Ambulatory Care and Insurance Coverage in an Era of Constraint

RONALD M. ANDERSEN, PH.D.
LU ANN ADAY, PH.D.
CHRISTOPHER S. LYTTLE, M.A.
LLEWELLYN J. CORNELIUS, M.A.
MEEI-SHIA CHEN, PH.D., M.P.H.

University of Chicago,
Center for Health Administration Studies
Continuing CHAS Research Series — No. 35

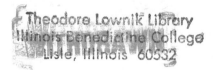

Pluribus Press, Inc.
Chicago

91 90 89 88 87   5 4 3 2 1

Library of Congress Catalog Card Number: 87-60398

International Standard Book Number: 0-931028-90-6

Pluribus Press, Inc., Division of Teach'em, Inc.
160 East Illinois Street
Chicago, IL 60611

Center for Health Administration Studies
University of Chicago
1101 East 58th Street, Suite 111
Chicago, IL 60637

Printed in the United States of America

Table of Contents

List of Tables and Figures

Foreword

IN 1972, The Robert Wood Johnson Foundation emerged as a national philanthropy devoted to improving the health and medical care of Americans. In addition to funding individual projects, a major share of its resources has been devoted to national initiatives. These have typically been five-year or longer multimillion-dollar demonstrations exploring the advantages of modifying the structure and organization of the health delivery system or changing professional education programs and technical and managerial practices of health practitioners, and of refining the ways health policies and programs are implemented. Many of these national initiatives were "tested" and refined first in small, one or two site pilot demonstrations.

During these years, the Foundation's overall program was designed in considerable part on the basis of a number of widely held beliefs, including: (1) that too many Americans were experiencing difficulties in obtaining front-line general or primary medical care; (2) that these deficiencies were found not only in low-income rural and urban inner city areas but also in many parts of more affluent urban and suburban America; (3) that these problems were related to inadequate out-of-hospital resources in many communities; and (4) that some of the shortfalls were due to an improper mix of physicians, with too many specialists and too few generalists.

A critical early step in the design of both the Foundation's overall program and particular intervention projects was to identify the extent of the problem to be attacked and the characteristics of the population needing the most assistance. When the Foundation initiated its grants program, it found that sufficient solid data on the overall "access to health care problems" were simply not available. A number of important questions could not be objectively answered. These included: How many Americans had a regular physician to whom they could go when ill or when they needed advice about their health? Was care reasonably convenient and affordable? Could individuals or groups who did not have a physician be identified and characterized? To acquire this type of information, the Foundation supported a series of baseline studies that measured the extent to which persons in the U.S. were experiencing problems in gaining access to desired medical care, and to what degree this was attributable to the absence of health resources or to imbalances in the mix of physician specialists and other health care professionals. These studies provided a yardstick against which to measure the later impact of a number of the Foundation's national initiatives to improve ambulatory care.

In this volume, *Ambulatory Care and Insurance Coverage in an Era of Constraint*, the Center for Health Administration Studies at the University of Chicago highlights some of the important public policy lessons learned from more than a decade of studies of a number of these large scale Foundation-public sector initiatives. These efforts sought to remedy the serious problems many Americans faced in obtaining continuing medical care when they were ill but not in need of hospitalization. Many of these studies were developed by the Center for Health Administration Studies, and represent some of the largest research efforts ever undertaken to assess the problems Americans face in obtaining medical care, and to evaluate the impact on these problems of major demonstrations of ways to improve the structure and organization of the health care system.

Readers of this work will discover that these many studies looked at together yield valuable insights into the nation's continuing access to care problems and produce some unexpected findings likely to be of important use to public policy makers working to improve our ways of delivering medical care.

ROBERT J. BLENDON

Senior Vice President
The Robert Wood Johnson Foundation

Executive Summary

T HIS BOOK discusses how recent changes in the organization and financing of medical care in the United States have affected access to medical care for the U.S. population as a whole and for traditionally disadvantaged subgroups within it. Two questions that emerge as particularly relevant as a result of these changes are:

1) What are the major differences in sources and financing of medical care for different segments of the U.S. population?

2) What impact do differences in sources and financing of care have on their actual access to medical care?

Five data sets were included in the analyses to address these questions — a 1982 national telephone survey, surveys of New York City and the poor in Arizona, and multi-site studies of a sample of eleven U.S. communities and five inner city areas in connection with evaluations of the Community Hospital Program (CHP) and Municipal Health Services Program (MHSP). These studies collected data between early 1981 and late 1982, with most of the interviews conducted in 1982. Because earlier questionnaires developed by the Center for Health Administration Studies were the basis for the design of many of the questions asked in these studies, there is a consistency in the availability and a considerable degree of comparability among data elements.

The analyses focus on describing regular sources of care and insurance coverage, and the characteristics of people with different sources and coverage. We then turn to the health care needs of people served by various sources and the impact of these sources on access to care. Then, using multivariate analysis, we model the process of obtaining a regular source of care and insurance coverage, as well as the special access problems and outcomes for people with different sources of care and coverage.

The study sites are diverse. The Arizona sample represents a very poor population and New York City an inner city minority population, as does the MHSP sample. The Community Hospital Program study sites more closely resemble the U.S. population as a whole, though some of the CHP communities also have large minority populations.

Most Americans use private doctors as their regular source of care. The low-income population in Arizona, New York City and the MHSP samples are, on the other hand, more likely to use hospital outpatient departments (OPDs) regularly. Of the approximately one out of ten people who do not have a regular source of care, many say they would go to a doctor's office or private clinic if they needed care. A third to a half could not name any place they would go. For most of those who do not have a regular source, the choice appears to be voluntary — they do not feel they need one, are seldom sick, or get care regularly but do not identify one particular place as their primary medical provider.

A closer look at the health care needs of this group confirms that people who do not have a regular source of care tend to have better health. Hospital OPD users, the publicly insured and the low-income — especially in the Arizona sample — had the poorest health status overall.

The vast majority of Americans have some type of private health insurance coverage. Public coverage is more important for the low-income and inner city populations. Many elderly have private coverage supplementary to Medicare. A very large proportion of the poor in Arizona (approximately one-third), where at the time of the survey no Medicaid program existed, reported having no insurance coverage. From 11 percent to 14 percent of the other samples reported being uninsured. A disproportionate number of these in all the studies were low-income.

People with a private doctor and some private health insurance are more likely to have higher incomes and educational levels and less likely to be members of a minority race than those people without any insurance coverage or a regular source. Though they represent a relatively small proportion of the total U.S. population (2 percent), the people who have no identifiable sources of care and coverage might be expected to have the greatest access problem.

Many of the traditional realized access differentials by race and income *per se* have disappeared, but where individuals go for care and whether they are insured do indeed continue to have an important impact. Regular hospital OPD users, for example, many of whom are publicly insured low-income minorities, tend to have less convenient care, lower rates of ambulatory care relative to their need, and more hospitalizations, but tend to pay less out of their own pockets for care. People with no insurance continue to have lower realized access rates, both overall and for illness-related and preventive reasons, than do either publicly or privately insured individuals.

Who appears to be most vulnerable to current changes underway in the U.S. health care system? People who use hospital OPDs as their regular source of care, especially those who only have some form of public insurance coverage or no insurance, are prime candidates for dumping or underservice in the increasingly constrained health care environment. Americans who do not have a regular source of medical care, particularly those in poor health who want one but can't afford it, should be of particular concern in emerging initiatives to develop managed systems of care for the indigent. The uninsured are least able to afford the high cost of medical care. The uninsured poor particularly tend to have the poorest health and it is these individuals who should receive special attention in efforts to cover the medically indigent who slip through the cracks of existing public and private systems of coverage.

These analyses confirm the importance of care and coverage as predictors of adequate access. These are the dimensions which are the focus of health policymaking regarding the organization and financing of care in the United States at the present time. The analyses reported here help identify the types of Americans who are most vulnerable to these changes. The book concludes with recommendations and suggestions for research to better inform the formulation of future policies affecting these groups.

Acknowledgments

THE AUTHORS gratefully acknowledge the support provided by the Robert Wood Johnson Foundation (Princeton, New Jersey) which has made this project possible.

Additionally, we are thankful for the support and stimulation of our colleagues at the Center for Health Administration Studies, the University of Chicago. Finally, we would like to thank Leah Schlesinger, Catherine Fay Glen, Myer Abraham Blank, and Christine Ostapiuk for contributing to the execution of the many data manipulation details of this research, and Annette Loretta Twells and Joyce Van Grondelle for competently typing the text and tables of this report.

RONALD ANDERSEN, Ph.D.
LU ANN ADAY, Ph.D.
CHRISTOPHER SHERMAN LYTTLE, M.A.
LLEWELLYN JOSEPH CORNELIUS, M.A.
MEEI-SHIA CHEN, Ph.D, M.P.H.

Introduction

MAJOR CHANGES are under way in the organization and financing of medical care in the United States. The number and kinds of HMOs and other primary care alternatives are increasing. Hospital inpatient utilization rates are declining. A variety of new preferred provider alternatives are being offered to the poor. Diagnosis Related Groups (DRGs) under Medicare have radically altered the system of the public financing of care for the elderly. Private insurers are becoming increasingly concerned about cost shifting and are beginning to forge selective contracts with providers to contain costs. Hospitals are becoming more and more concerned about the level of uncompensated care they provide, and consumers about the increasing share of health care costs they are paying out of their own pockets. A cost containment oriented congress promises to reduce the level of support for many health and human services programs over the next few years.

These changes are hypothesized to portend profound changes for access to medical care in the United States, particularly on the part of those groups and individuals most affected by major policy developments — the poor, the uninsured, those with some form of public third-party coverage, and people who have tended to use hospital outpatient services for their regular source of care. The proportion of the poor covered under Medicaid is declining. Economic-related "transfers" are presumably increasing in many hospitals. Many providers are becoming more wary of taking on public pay patients. Increased consumer co-payments and deductibles will probably lead to lower utilization rates, but the resultant effect on access to *needed* services remains unclear.

The Robert Wood Johnson Foundation has sponsored major national and community surveys that provide a wealth of information on the state of the nation and representative local areas with respect to access to medical care. The analyses of these data reported here for a 1982 national telephone survey of the U.S. population, the poor of the State of Arizona, the population of New York City with a special oversample of the poor in that city, surveys of twelve diverse communities in connection with the Community Hospital Program evaluation, and of five inner city areas in the Municipal Health Services Program evaluation serve to illuminate the types of communities and individuals most apt to be affected by the changes currently underway in existing systems of care and coverage in the United States.

Chapter 1
Organizational and Financial Dimensions of Health Policy

LU ANN ADAY
LLEWELLYN J. CORNELIUS
RONALD M. ANDERSEN

THE HISTORY of health care in the United States reflects a gradual development of a variety of organizational structures and financial mechanisms for meeting consumer needs. The extent to which the needs of various groups have been met has been dependent upon both the type of medical services available to them, and the extent to which the financial burden has been diminished by public and/or third-party coverage for services. The current system of health care can be seen as a product of the evolution of the organizational and financial mechanisms in response to historical and current health policy developments.

The emergence of the current U.S. health care system has been characterized by Anderson as falling into roughly three periods: a period preceding 1930 in which the basic infrastructure for the current health care system was developed with the advent of the modern hospital and trained medical personnel; a second period from 1930-65, characterized in particular by the growth of major public and private mechanisms for the financing of care; and a third period since 1965, which has been concerned with trying to manage and control the "monster" wrought by the developments of the first two periods. In particular, there has been a concern since the mid-1960s with the resultant skyrocketing costs of care and *new* organization and financing mechanisms that might be implemented to contain seemingly inexorable increases (Anderson, 1985).

Throughout each of these periods, parallel but distinct tiers of care and financing have been available to different groups. The Great Society initiatives of the early 1960s were intended to reduce many of these inequities. A profound concern with the present cost-containment policy initiatives is that the disadvantaged who have achieved the greatest gain through prior public policy may well be the most vulnerable to the current efforts to contain costs.

This chapter (1) presents an analytic framework, which will serve to guide our analyses of the groups most vulnerable to these changes in health policy, and (2) trace the roots of these current organizational and financial developments, with particular attention to the different tiers of caring and paying for care and their vulnerability to the changing tides of health policy.

Health Policy Vulnerability Framework

Health policy has been the starting point for much of the conceptual work in formalizing what is meant by "access" (Aday and Andersen, 1974; Aday and Andersen, 1975; Aday, et al., 1980; Aday, et al., 1984). Changes in the organization and financing of medical care are hypothesized to have a major impact on the potential and realized access to services. Figure 1.1 provides an analytic framework for constructing a policy vulnerability profile of who is most apt to be impacted by these changes, which will guide the analyses that follow. The basic categories of variables are based on a behavioral model of health services utilization and access (Andersen, 1968).

Policy vulnerability refers to the extent to which the potential or actual access of different groups may be influenced by changes in the organization and financing of care. The dimensions to consider are those which may suggest *potential* vulnerability to developments, as well as *actual* problems in obtaining access to care. The dimensions of potential vulnerability refer to target groups that may be differentially impacted by the focus of particular policies, e.g., the elderly by Medicare, the poor by Medicaid, residents of rural or inner city areas by manpower programs, the medically needy by certain program eligibility criteria, etc. The proof of the effectiveness of these policies is whether access may *ultimately* be affected as a result of different "means" being available to these groups. The regular source of care and insurance

Figure 1.1. Analytic Model for Health Policy Vulnerability

DIMENSIONS OF POLICY VULNERABILITY	CATEGORIES OF BEHAVIORAL MODEL				
	Predisposing →	Need →	Enabling →	Utilization →	Satisfaction
Potential Selection	Age Sex Education Occupation Ethnicity				
			Income		
Need		Perceived Health Disability Days			
System			Residence Region Supply Ratios Community Per Capita Income		
Means			Regular Source Insurance Coverage		
Actual Access			Convenience	Contact Volume Type of Service Expenditures	Satisfaction

coverage variables are the focal point of the vulnerability question. A variety of predisposing, enabling, and need variables may be predictive of who has what kind of care and coverage. The proof of the import of these factors is the actual convenience, utilization of, and satisfaction with care resulting from having or not having particular types of providers or insurance.

Selection refers to those correlates which are predictive of whether individuals want or may be targeted to receive a certain type of care or coverage. These dimensions are immutable to health policy *per se*, but are important descriptors of who has what kind of provider and insurance, and who may, therefore, have the most and least to lose by a reorientation of existing policies.

Need refers to indicators of those who require care the most. From a needs-oriented perspective on equity, it is those in need who are most "deserving" of care. Of particular concern here is how need may vary for those who have different "means" (regular source and insurance) of access available. Those with the most need, but the fewest resources (e.g., no insurance and/or no regular provider), may be potentially the most vulnerable to policies that exacerbate or fail to eliminate these barriers.*

The system dimension refers to the characteristics of the health care environment in which an individual resides. This dimension refers to aggregate system-level descriptors of the organization and financing of care in an area. It embodies indicators which are most apt to register area-wide changes in the availability or distribution of health care resources, e.g., supply to population ratios, mean per capita income.

The means dimension refers to the most immediate operational indicators for how the individual patient's care is organized and financed — whether one has or does not have and/or the type of regular source of care or insurance coverage. It is the most immediate expression for the individual of the health care policy-oriented organizational and financial resources potentially available to enhance access.

Access is the ultimate outcome of how services are organized and financed. It may be viewed from a more process-oriented point of view, for instance, by the convenience of services, or a more objective or subjective outcome-oriented perspective, as represented by indicators of utilization and satisfaction. All of the preceding factors may be said to contribute to this ultimate access outcome.

The most immediate policy-relevant dimension, an individual's regular source of care and insurance coverage, will be the

---

*In the original behavioral model, need is viewed as subsequent to enabling conditions and the most immediate or direct cause of utilization. For this analysis we feel it is better to consider need prior to enablement since we are particularly interested in the selection of patients with varying needs into different kinds of regular care sources.

focal point of the analyses to be undertaken here. We will explore who is most likely to have what type of care and coverage, how system characteristics seem to impact their choices, what are the relative needs of these individuals, and ultimately the influence of having different types of care and coverage on access to medical care.

Policy vulnerability analysis may be seen as the consideration of the extent to which different groups may be differentially influenced in the choices and outcomes of how their care is organized and financed by changes in health policy. We will, in particular, focus on who is most likely to be impacted by current policy developments, what their needs are, how satisfactory their access seems to be, and how they might be affected by these developments. The framework introduced here and operationalized in the analyses that follow is intended to illuminate the groups most vulnerable to shifts in health policy historically and currently as the decade of constraint in the U.S. health care system deepens.

Organization of Care

Historical Policy Developments

Originally, private physicians were the primary source of medical care for the U.S. population. Physician services were provided either in a patient's home, or in almshouses and public dispensaries, depending on whether the patient was wealthy or poor (Williams, 1984: 136). The almshouses that were built by local governments, the voluntary hospitals built by charitable organizations, and public dispensaries were the principal sources of medical care for the poor. The voluntary hospital only cared for those who were classified as "the worthy poor," leaving the unworthy poor, along with the incurable and chronically ill, to rely on the almshouse for medical care (Rosenberg, 1982; Starr, 1982). Other social classes were reluctant to use the voluntary hospitals, both because of the proliferation of diseases, as well as the possible stigma attached to using them (Hartwell, 1975: 12).

After the improvement of medical care through the introduction of antiseptic surgery (Starr, 1982: 155; Anderson and Gevitz, 1983: 309; Anderson, 1984: 68-69), all social classes began to rely more on hospitals for medical care. The system of hospitals that developed at this time included the voluntary hospital, the public hospitals (particularly those supported by municipal governments), and hospitals sponsored by ethnic or religious groups, developed to counter discrimination in voluntary hospitals (Starr, 1982: 173).

Despite the expansion in this period preceding the Depression, the Committee on the Costs of Medical Care reported that only 47 percent of the families surveyed received the services of a physician during the course of a year, 21 percent had seen a dentist, and only 5.9 percent had any sort of hospital care (Falk, et al., 1933: 63). The Committee also found that "the percentage of individuals who obtain no medical service is greater the lower the family income, ranging from slightly less than 14 percent among those in families with incomes of $10,000 or more, to nearly 50 percent for those families less than $1,200" (Falk, et al., 1933: 69). The Committee also concluded that although the Black American family was not systematically studied, it could be safely assumed that they were receiving less medical care than the lowest income group in the study (i.e., < $1,200 and between $1,200 and $2,000) (Committee on the Costs of Medical Care, 1932: 10).

After World War II in 1946 the Hospital Survey and Construction (Hill-Burton) Act was passed in an effort to improve the access to medical care for the entire population by increasing the nation's supply of hospital beds. It did, in fact, succeed in increasing the number of beds from around 3.2 per 1,000 to over its targeted number of 4.5 per 1,000 (NCHS, 1984; 1985). However, since the act required that the sponsoring group provide two-thirds of the funds for the hospital's construction, many poor and rural communities were not able to obtain funding for their projects (Thompson, 1981: 35; Starr, 1982: 350). Though there were requirements for funded hospitals to provide "community service" and "free care", they were not well-enforced. A separate-but-equal clause for some facilities in the South continued to sanction patterns of racial segregation (President's Commission, 1983).

Concern about the availability of physicians led, after World War II, to increased federal support for medical education. There was, in particular, concern about the numbers of generalists and practitioners who would serve in rural and urban inner city areas, and the lack of minority and female physicians. The most direct federal support for medical education began with the Health Professions Educational Assistance Act of 1963 and subsequent amendments. Evidence shows that it and other direct affirmative action programs succeeded in increasing the number of physicians, as well as the number of minority and women providers, but that it did not necessarily succeed in redistributing large numbers of them to the areas of greatest need (Lewis, et al., 1976; President's Commission, 1983).

The major federal initiatives aimed at the provision and reorganization of services to serve the disadvantaged were those of the Johnson administration's Great Society Program. The Neighborhood Health Center and National Health Service Corps programs were directly concerned with placing providers in medically underserved areas. Evidence indicates that the Neighborhood Health Centers did succeed in enhancing access and reducing infant mortality rates in the poor communities in which they were established, while maintaining reasonably priced care. They did, however, require a considerable federal subsidy to survive—a commitment which was erratically provided by successive administrations. The National Health Service Corps is credited with placing physicians in areas of need on a short-term basis, but did not appear to be successful in enlisting large numbers of providers in those areas to practice (President's Commission, 1983).

Public hospitals were most often providers of "last resort" for the poor who had no means to pay. Community and university *teaching* hospitals provided large amounts of "free" medical care to the indigent through their outpatient and inpatient teaching programs. Through the years public *and* community hospital outpatient departments (OPDs) and emergency rooms (ERs) increasingly became major providers of primary care (Bryant, et al., 1976).

In the early 1970s this trend came to be viewed as a crisis by many in the health care field. Concern was expressed that hospitals should consider (1) the impact of the large amounts of frontline primary care being provided through their OPDs and ERs, and (2) what new organizational arrangements needed to be created to coordinate these services, improve their financial and managerial efficiency, and enhance the access of the populations traditionally served in these settings (Bryant, et al., 1976; Goldsmith, 1977).

In the early 1970s the Robert Wood Johnson Foundation responded with the Community Hospital Program (CHP), to rationalize the role of hospitals in the provision of front-line primary care. The CHP provided approximately $27 million in grant funds to over 50 community hospitals to initiate hospital-sponsored primary care group practices. It represented one of the largest private sector initiatives in support of the organization of primary care services in the United States (Shortell, et al., 1984; Aday, et al., 1985). In the late 1970s the Foundation attempted to extend a comparable model to public hospitals through its Municipal Health Services Program (MHSP). The MHSP encouraged municipal hospital systems to develop primary-care oriented clinics to better serve the poor and the elderly clients of the public hospitals in five participating cities (Fleming and Andersen, 1986). These innovations did seem to enhance access without increasing the cost of care to the target populations. In the analyses to be reported later in this book, data from large-scale social survey evaluations conducted in the target areas served by the CHP and MHSP sites will be used to further examine who would have the most to gain or lose by subsequent efforts to expand or curtail programs of this kind.

In the 1970s, in an effort to deal with what was perceived to be a pending crisis in the system resulting from the rapidly rising costs of care, new organizational strategies were introduced in the public sector as well. Some were more regulatory in focus and others more competition-oriented.

In 1973 President Nixon signed the HMO Act into law. This HMO "innovation" had its roots in the concept of prepaid medical groups introduced by the Committee on the Costs of Medical Care in the early 1930s and expressed in early forms of organization, such as Group Health Plan in Washington, D.C., Health Insurance Plan (HIP) of New York and the Kaiser Permanente Health Plan in California (Anderson, 1985). The HMO concept, however, combined the financing and delivery mechanisms and encouraged the reduction of unnecessary utilization and costs through prevention and cost-effective oriented care. Initially HMOs primarily enrolled employee groups and the middle class. There were few or no mechanisms for the unemployed, uninsured, or publicly insured to participate in these plans.

In this same period the National Health Planning and Resources Development Act (1974) was passed. This act was concerned with regulating the expansion of new health care facilities, to contain what was seen as an inflation-fueling growth of the health care system. The principal mechanisms enacted were a federal mandate of certificate-of-need laws in each state and the establishment of health systems planning agencies to regulate the construction and/or expansion of facilities. Evaluations of certificate-of-need programs indicated that they did not reduce the overall level of investment in facilities and services, and that the political nature of the decision making in many agencies resulted in the more powerful, rather than the less powerful, benefitting in many communities (President's Commission, 1983).

Recent Policy Developments

The discussion of major historical policy developments in the organization of medical care has suggested variant patterns of success in improving the availability of services to all tiers of American society. Since 1980, most of these initiatives have been subject to large-scale shifts in philosophical and/or financial support by the Reagan administration.

The legislation to increase the numbers of physicians did succeed quite well. The number of M.D.s doubled from around 260,000 in 1960 to 520,000 in 1983 (AMA, 1985; U.S. Bureau of the Census, 1985). In 1980, a prestigious national commission — the Graduate Medical Education National Advisory Committee (GMENAC) — found that there were too many, rather than not enough, physicians and that this "surplus" would become even larger by the end of the decade (GMENAC, 1981).

The Reagan administration's position on medical manpower and medical education built directly on these GMENAC findings. It has sought to eliminate all funding for health manpower training programs supported under Title VII of the Public Health Service Act. Congress has fought to keep aspects of these programs, particularly to direct support more narrowly to economically disadvantaged students and to reduce the government's potential losses resulting from non-payment of loans under the Health Education Assistance Loan (HEAL) program. Iglehart notes that the "current Title VII health manpower programs do not encourage the education of more physicians, but rather provide support for narrowly defined purposes that Congress has previously deemed in the public interest" (Iglehart, 1986: 328). This serves as quite a contrast to the aggressive and expansive federal policy in support of medical education in the early 1970s.

Explicit affirmative action programs for minorities have diminished as well. Evidence indicates that minority physicians are more apt to serve minority and Medicaid patients, and practice in underserved areas. Cutbacks in federal support for medical education in general and affirmative action in particular may result in a diminished number of physicians available to serve the disadvantaged (Keith, et al., 1985; Shea and Fullilove, 1985).

The Reagan administration has also sought to eliminate or substantially reduce support for Community Health Centers (CHCs) and the National Health Services Corps. In 1982 the administration attempted to incorporate the CHCs into a primary care block grant to allow the states more power to decide whether particular centers would be maintained. Correspondingly this reduced the overall budget for these initiatives by a third. The Congress has continued to maintain the categorical status of CHCs, but allocations have not kept pace with inflation. The administration also sought to eliminate all support for the National Health Service Corps. Thus far the Congress has maintained some minimal level of support, but has encouraged the linkage of Corps physicians to organized practice settings, such as the CHCs (American Public Health Association, 1985).

We saw earlier that the CHCs were apparently successful in improving access and achieving lower rates of infant mortality in many low income communities. Administration opposition, lukewarm Congressional support, and even more dramatic cutbacks implied in the Gramm-Rudman budget balancing legislation raise doubts that these previous gains will be maintained, much less enhanced.

Public and community hospitals continue to be major providers of front-line primary care. Of increasing concern, however, are the large amounts of uncompensated charity and bad debt care which these hospitals (particularly public hospitals) are being forced to assume (Sloan, et al., 1986). Public hospitals have traditionally provided disproportionately more "free" care, because of the large number of poor they serve. There is a concern that more constrained reimbursement for public pay (Medicare and Medicaid) patients will result in larger financial burdens for these institutions. Evidence also shows increased "economic transfers" of the uninsured as a result of the tendency for voluntary and for-profit hospitals to "dump" these or other patients they would prefer to "get-out-of-my-emergency-room" (GOMERs) to public facilities (Leiderman and Grisso, 1985; Schiff, et al., 1986). Public institutions' care of the uninsured is increasingly the subject of debate. These debates focus on how the burden of caring for the poor should be more fairly distributed and how this care can be financially viable in the long run.

The CHP was demonstrated to be effective in improving access to medical care in many communities. It seemed to offer a viable alternative to enhancing front-line primary care services under the auspices of community hospitals committed to developing such alternatives. An evaluation of the CHP concluded that the development of these alternatives might best be enhanced by loan guarantees to interested hospitals, particularly those with fewer resources or serving large numbers of the disadvantaged (Shortell, et al., 1984; Aday et al., 1985). Currently a climate of constraint at the federal level is unlikely to enable the provision of such subsidies, however. The subsequent development of such a model will be largely dependent on the financial resources available through the institution itself or the community it serves. This is unlikely to enhance the availability of such alternatives in poor neighborhoods, which seemed to benefit most from the Johnson Foundation-funded groups.

Similarly the Municipal Health Services Program assumed an external subsidy. Financially strapped public hospital systems are less likely to start practices of this kind on their own (Fleming and Andersen, 1986).

The number and kinds of HMOs and other prepaid alternatives have accelerated in recent years with the growth of for-profit health care and the increasing horizontal and vertical integration of the health care system (Goldsmith, 1981). Increasing federal efforts are being made to encourage the enrollment of the poor and elderly in a variety of prepaid and managed care systems (Altman, 1983). Evidence indicates that utilization and costs may well be lower as a result of being in a prepaid system of care (Luft, 1981). Whether access and quality will be better in these settings remains unanswered. The Reagan administration has sought to eliminate all formal health planning efforts. The spirit of competition, not regulation, characterizes the Reagan administration's policy on how health care services should be organized and managed (American Public Health Association, 1985).

Financing of Care

The Depression marked the beginning of both some initiative on the part of the government to absorb the cost of care for the poor, as well as the introduction of voluntary health insurance as a mechanism for mediating the cost for the employed in particular. Originating with the Blue Cross and Blue Shield (Starr, 1982: 295-310; Anderson, 1984: 71), voluntary plans provided insurance for the members of the workforce who were either able to purchase the insurance outright through their employer, or have the cost paid as a benefit.

Historical Policy Developments

Concrete expression of public support for coverage for the poor and elderly began with Social Security in the mid-1930s. Subsequently, encouragement was provided to the states to issue vouchers to the medically indigent and elderly who might not qualify under categoric cash assistance programs. The culmination of federal involvement in the financing of care was the enactment of the Medicaid and Medicare programs for the poor and elderly in 1965 (Anderson, 1985).

The primary role of the federal government in the implementation of the Medicare program was to pay the providers for rendering services to the elderly. The fee-for-service method of reimbursing providers was fully maintained. The government allocated the administration of the program to a fiscal intermediary of the hospitals', extended care facilities', and home health services providers' choosing. The majority of the groups chose Blue Cross for Medicare Part A, and Blue Shield for Medicare Part B (Starr, 1982: 375). "As a result, the administration of Medicare was lodged in the private insurance systems originally established to suit provider interests, and the federal government surrendered direct control of its program and costs" (Starr, 1982: 375).

The Medicaid program represented an expansion of previous federal/state initiatives for the provision of medical care for the poor (U.S.D.H.E.W., 1975: 6-7). In the Medicaid program states were given both the option to participate and to decide which services over and above a set minimally required to provide for its clients (U.S.D.H.E.W., 1975: 7). Besides not having direct control over the Medicare program and its costs, the federal government did not have direct control over the Medicaid program as a whole, since the role of implementing was left to the states. Considerable diversity in the range and extent of covered services evolved. One state (Arizona) did not develop a Medicaid-type program until very recently. In the analyses to follow, the particular access problems of the poor in Arizona, prior to this program, will be examined.

Although Medicaid was meant to improve access to medical care for the poor, Starr explains that when the Medicaid program began in 1965, it "omitted from coverage most two-parent families, and childless couples, widows, and other single persons under the age of sixty-five years, families with fathers working at low paying jobs, and the medically needy in twenty-two states that did not provide coverage" (Starr, 1982: 374). Nonetheless, as a result of the organizational and financial efforts of the Great Society programs, "83 percent of all families had some health insurance coverage in 1970 — up 20 percentage points from 1953 and 9 percentage points from 1963" (Andersen, et al., 1976: 110). Further, the utilization rates of the traditionally poor and disadvantaged increased and gaps between the poor and nonpoor began to diminish or disappear (Aday, et al., 1984).

This enhanced access was not without its price. The cost of these programs continued to rise. The federal share of health care expenditures tripled from 10.1 percent in 1965 to 29.6 percent in 1984 (NCHS, 1985). An all-time high proportion of the gross national product (over ten percent) was being spent on health care by 1982 (NCHS, 1985). Predictions in the early 1980s were that the Health Insurance Trust Fund, which provided funds for Medicare, would be bankrupt by 1990 (Congressional Budget Office, 1983). Early in the decade, the Reagan administration acted to make dramatic changes in the Medicare and Medicaid programs, in an effort to avert a major financial crisis in these programs.

Recent Policy Developments

The Omnibus Budget Reconciliation Act of 1981 moved towards designing a financing system that was based on a prospective payment system for hospital services rendered to Medicare eligible patients (Lohr and Marquis, 1984). The Tax Equity and Fiscal

Responsibility Act of 1982 established the basis for such a system, which was enacted through the diagnosis-related method of reimbursement (DRGs) in the Social Security Amendments of 1983.

> Under DRGs, a price is set prospectively for each type of case or illness. Everything that could be done to hospital patients was divided into 467 categories, each with a fixed price set by computing what similar types of hospitals had been charging for similar cases. Revenues would not vary with what the hospital actually did (Morone and Dunham, 1984: 81).

The implementation of a prospective payment system under Medicare was a major and fundamental change in the basis for reimbursing services (Lohr and Marquis, 1984). The Omnibus Deficit Reduction Act of 1984 froze Medicare reimbursement for physician fees and reduced increases in the DRG rates for hospitals. Corresponding to the constraints and reductions in the levels of reimbursement for providers are legislated increases in the levels of coinsurance and deductibles charged to consumers under both Parts A and B of the program. The deductibles for Part A have increased from $40 in 1966 to $144 in 1978, and finally to an average of $520 per hospital stay in 1987 (Aday and Andersen, 1981: 22; HCFA 1987). The Reagan administration has also proposed some other major modifications to Medicare, such as the provision of vouchers to recipients for the purchase of private coverage in the marketplace, and catastrophic coverage for enrollees through an increase in the Part B premium. Considerable concern has been expressed about the probable equity implications resulting from increased cost-sharing by elderly Medicare patients, the willingness of providers to serve these clients resulting from lower levels of reimbursement, and the issue of premature discharge, with inadequate post-discharge care arrangements (Dolenc and Dougherty, 1985; Newcomer, et al., 1985; Spiegel and Kavaler, 1985).

The Omnibus Budget Reconciliation Act of 1981 had its major impact on Medicaid—the principal financing program for the poor. It legislated successive reductions in federal funding at the rate of 3 percent in fiscal year 1982, 4 percent in 1983 and 4.5 percent in 1984 (Altman, 1983). The states would have to decide how much of the burden for Medicaid they would begin to assume, given successive federal reductions over the next five years (*Health Care Financial Management*, 1986: 5-7).

In addition to successive reductions in the overall level of federal support for Medicaid the categories of individuals eligible for Medicaid have been constricted; the free choice of provider has been waived, enabling states to develop innovative arrangements for enrolling Medicaid-eligibles with preferred providers or case-management oriented primary care networks; and the amount which consumers may have to pay out-of-pocket for certain optional, as well as mandatory, services has been increased (Altman, 1983; Mundinger, 1985).

Recent statistics show that the number of Medicaid recipients declined over the period of these federal cutbacks from 22,831,000 in 1977 to around 21,808,000 in 1985 (HCFA, 1986). To find the extent to which Medicaid reaches the poor one looks at the ratio of the total number of Medicaid recipients reported by HCFA over time to the total number of individuals below 125 percent of the poverty level. The proportion of the poor and near poor covered by Medicaid reached a peak of around 64 percent in the mid 1970s and has subsequently declined to about 47 percent by 1984 (*Health Care Financing Review*, 1985; HCFA, 1986; U.S. Bureau of the Census, 1986). Cutbacks seem to have had an impact on the relative "proportion" of the poor actually served under Medicaid.

Physicians have also reacted to the adjustment in reimbursement rates for Medicare and Medicaid patients by being less willing to treat these patients (Gabel and Rice, 1985: 605-606). Some of the expected consequences of discouragement of utilization of the medical system are decreases in the amount of medical care received by disadvantaged people (Davis and Rowland, 1983: 160). Some patients may defer treatment since they can not afford it (Aday, et al., 1984: 85), and the health of the poor and elderly will be adversely affected as a result (Mundinger, 1985).

Due to the recent changes in the financing of medical care it has been estimated that in 1983 about 29.2 million people had no health insurance. This reflects an increase in the percentage of the nation's uninsured from around 9 to 10 percent in 1976 to 12 to 15 percent at the present time (Iglehart, 1985: 59-60). This group of uninsured is comprised of two sub-groups: those who are always uninsured, and those who are sometimes uninsured "The always uninsured are individuals without Medicare, Medicaid, or private insurance coverage for the entire year . . . the sometimes uninsured are those who were covered by public or private insurance part of the year, but were uninsured the remainder of the year" (Davis and Rowland, 1983: 151-152).

Part of the group of the permanently uninsured appears to be those who have lost their jobs. As Berki, et al. conclude, one's place of employment previously provided health insurance for most of 1,332 unemployed individuals in the Detroit area (Berki, et al., 1985: 849-851). Another part of the permanently uninsured group has developed from the recent cutbacks of Medicaid beneficiaries described earlier. The cutbacks for Medicare beneficiaries have focused more on increasing the costs of deductibles, than on trimming the pool of eligible participants.

In some ways an era of constraint has just begun. To curb the federal deficit on December 12, 1985, President Reagan signed the Gramm-Rudman-Hollings bill. This law required that the federal deficit be eliminated using conventional legislative means or, if that failed, through automatic spending cuts over a five–year period. Some health care and welfare programs, particularly those relating to service provision for the poor, were presumably "exempt" from "automatic" cuts. These included Medicaid; Aid to Families with Dependent Children (AFDC); Women, Infants, and Children (WIC) program; food stamps; and child nutrition. This exemption simply meant these programs were exempt from the Reagan administration's across-the-board cutting. Congress and the administration, in the context of their regular budget reconciliation process, could make whatever cuts they thought appropriate to meet the deficit reduction goals (*Congressional Quarterly*, 1985).

The automatic cutting aspect of the bill has been ruled unconstitutional. It does, however, continue to provide a framework for the Congress to apply in reducing the federal deficit.

All of this serves to indicate major changes in the organization and financing of care that have been underway in recent years; and the large and direct impact these changes have had on the availability and modes of delivery and coverage of the population for the high cost of illness. One can expect that concerned providers and payers may have to make some major adaptations if they wish to control the cost — without jeopardizing the access — to quality care for the groups most vulnerable to these developments.

Summary

This chapter has presented a health policy-oriented framework for considering the impact of major changes in the organization and financing of care on access. Of particular concern was a consideration of historical and recent health policy developments and who might be most vulnerable to these changes. The framework, which will serve to guide the analyses that follow, identified characteristics of individuals and the health care system that signal who they are, what types of care and coverage they have, and how changes in the organization and financing of services might impact upon their ultimate access to services in an era of deepening constraints in the U.S. health care system.

Summary

Chapter 2
Empirical and Methodological Studies of Care and Coverage

LLEWELLYN J. CORNELIUS

LU ANN ADAY

THE TRENDS previously discussed suggest that organization and financing factors have greatly influenced the extent to which certain policy vulnerable groups have been able to gain access to medical care. Yet empirical studies on the organization and financing of care do not always provide one with conclusive evidence concerning the nature of this relationship.

For example, Mechanic notes in his review of several multivariate studies of the utilization of medical care that health status explained the largest amount of variation in the utilization of health services in these models (Andersen, et al., 1975; Hershey, et al., 1975; Kohn and White, 1976; Andersen and Aday, 1978; Wolinsky, 1978). He also found that a smaller amount of the variation was explained by the respondent's regular source of care and insurance coverage and an even smaller amount was due to factors such as age, income, ethnicity, and the education of the head of the family (Mechanic, 1979). On the other hand, Aday, et al. found that even after one adjusted for age, sex, and reported disability days, having a regular source of care and insurance were still significant predictors of seeing a physician during a given year (Aday, et al., 1984: 67). In this chapter we will look at other literature that seems to speak to the importance of these indicators — that we hope to examine in considerable detail both descriptively and analytically in the chapters to follow — and some of the methodological issues that might contribute to these variant findings.

Regular Source of Care

In terms of the importance that having a regular source of care plays in the use of medical care Berki and Ashcraft found that not only was the number of chronic visits and acute conditions shown to be the most consistent and powerful predictor of illness-related visits to physicians, but that not having a usual source of care was associated with fewer visits both for individuals and families (Berki and Ashcraft, 1979: 1177). Wan and Gray found in their study of 2,063 individuals living in five urban areas that having a regular source of care was significant in the utilization of preventive medical services. They also found that:

> Having a regular source of care was found to be related to social class, private insurance status and race, with higher-status individuals and whites most frequently using physicians. . . Moreover, those with no regular source of care had the most variability in sources of services and the lowest rate of utilization (Wan and Gray, 1978: 321).

Several researchers have concluded that not only does having a regular source of care affect the use of medical services, but having a particular doctor at that source contributes to the kind of medical care used. Wilensky and Rossiter noted that though 61 percent of all ambulatory visits in 1977 were initiated by the patients, over a third (39 percent) were initiated by their physician (Wilensky and Rossiter, 1983: 261). Physician discretion was greater in ambulatory versus surgery and hospital care. There was also greater discretion evident in the rates of expenditures for services, including those for X-rays and laboratory tests, compared to visits (Wilensky and Rossiter, 1983: 270). Berki and Ashcraft found that private practice physicians in general tend to use the hospitals less than HMO-based physicians (Berki and Ashcraft, 1979: 1173). Marcus and Stone on the other hand found that HMO patients who had a regular doctor used more physician services than those of a comparable fee-for-service group (Marcus and Stone, 1984: 653-4).

Berki and Ashcraft found that those that did not identify a regular doctor at their source of care (either an HMO or a physician's private practice) used more ambulatory care for a given hospitalization than a person who had a regular doctor (Berki and Ashcraft, 1979: 1172). Davidson documented that low-income, inner city residents used emergency departments as a substitute for not having a regular doctor, whereas others used this source "when their family doctors were not available" (Davidson, 1978: 131). This suggests that many low-income inner-city residents do not have ties with a regular doctor and as a result may receive more fragmented care than other groups. Schneider and Dove noted that high users of emergency departments in Veterans Administration hospitals tend to be people who have used ERs previously, have chronic disease, especially cardiovascular disease and chronic pulmonary disease, live near the hospital, and frequently use their specialty clinics (Schneider and Dove, 1983: 61). Thus there appears a variation in the use of medical care by whether or not the patient has a regular source of care, the type of place they go to, and whether the person has a particular provider at that source.

Sharp, et al. discovered that people who had positive attitudes about visiting physicians are more likely to consider symptoms serious enough to warrant a physician visit (Sharp, et al., 1983: 259). Likewise, Crandall and Duncan found that belief in the effectiveness of medical care increased the likelihood of poor patients having a physician contact as well as having a physical examination (Crandall and Duncan, 1981: 67, 69).

Linn, et al. concluded that there was greater patient satisfaction in settings where they did not have to wait long to see a health professional and where there was a greater amount of time spent by the health professionals with the patient than on administrative busy work. They also found that patient and physician satisfaction were greater in areas where the "charges for a routine follow-up visit are more realistic (using local Medicare prevailing rates as a standard)" (Linn, et al., 1985: 1177).

Goldberg and Dietrich determined that physicians' training history was not a major determinant of the quality of care they provided and subspecialists were just as likely as generalists to provide a high degree of continuity of care for their patients (Goldberg and Dietrich, 1985: 70). Kosecoff, et al. noted that patients seen in the group practices of fifteen teaching hospitals had a more favorable attitude towards the care they received than those surveyed in the 1976 National Access Study conducted by the Center for Health Administration Studies. They also report that these patients were often seen promptly upon arrival and that they generally saw the same provider (Kosecoff, 1985: 252-254). These studies suggest that the characteristics of providers as well as the patients' perceptions of their regular source are important in determining their ultimate utilization of and satisfaction with services.

Insurance Coverage

As in the case of the empirical studies on the regular source of care there is also a variety of studies conducted which examine the importance of insurance coverage in enabling the use of medical care. For example, Mitchell and Shurman found when comparing the reimbursement levels for Medicaid and Blue-Shield patients, that physicians were more willing to treat the Medicaid patients if their reimbursement levels were closer to that of the Blue-Shield patients (Mitchell and Shurman, 1984: 1030-31). Yelin, et al. found that when one holds medical symptoms and demographic variables constant individuals that lack health insurance coverage had fewer hospitalizations per year (Yelin, et al., 1983: 570).

Several recent studies have looked more closely at the relationship between private insurance coverage and the use of medical care. The Rand Health Insurance Study found that those assigned to an experimental group who received free care were more likely to have a physician visit, more hospital admissions, and more days of hospitalization than those assigned to a prepaid group practice (Newhouse, et al., 1981: 1504; Enthoven, 1984: 1528). Likewise, Wilensky and Rossiter found that when one varies the amount that a patient pays out of pocket for health insurance there is also a variation in the amount of medical care used — the higher the out-of-pocket cost, the fewer services that are utilized (Wilensky and Rossiter, 1983: 265). Lerner, et al. concluded that when Blue Cross extended their insurance coverage to outpatient services there was a decrease in inpatient admissions for the Blue Cross plan members (Lerner, et al., 1983: 107).

Wilensky, et al. found in looking at the variation in insurance coverage for the respondents under sixty-five in the National Medical Care Expenditures Study (NMCES) that 32 percent of all employees with premiums below $1,000 (for families and $400 for individuals—59 percent of the respondents) did not have semi-private room coverage; 9 percent of this same group had to pay a hospital deductible and 2 percent had no hospital coverage. On the other hand, the other 41 percent of the sample (i.e., those with premiums above $1,000 for families and $400 for individuals) were "less likely to have hospital and physician benefits with cost-sharing requirements. Only 18 percent did not have daily benefits covering the full costs of a semi-private hospital room, ignoring deductibles" (Wilensky, et al., 1984: 63). These studies show considerable variation in the amount and type of insurance coverage related to premiums paid. The variation in turn represents the degree of financial barriers people face in obtaining medical care.

Unlike some of the private insurance packages offered to employees, the Medicare program "was never expected to pay for all medical care expenditures of the elderly" (Cafferata, 1985: 1087). Thus some elderly patients over the years have purchased supplemental medical insurance in order to help bridge this gap in coverage (Cafferata, 1985: 1087). The Baucus legislation has been proposed in an effort to examine the adequacy of this supplemental insurance coverage. The legislation proposes that these packages cover the following at a minimum:

> co-payments for hospital days through the Medicare lifetime reserve (under Medicare's Hospital Insurance (Part A), benefits for 60 additional hospital days that can be used whenever a beneficiary has exhausted the 90 days in a covered benefit period), 90% coverage of all Medicare eligible hospital expenses for an additional 365 days after exhaustion of Medicare benefits, and coverage of the Medicare Part B 20% co-insurance, subject to a maximum deductible of $200 and a maximum benefit of no less than $5,000; a policy is not required to cover the Part A deductible, although nearly all do (Cafferata, 1985: 1088).

Using the standards set by the Baucus legislation as an index of the quality of medical plans for the elderly, Cafferata found that only 20 percent of the elderly sample respondents in the 1977 NMCES study had plans which met all the above requirements. It was also found that "it was more common to find coverage for inpatient than outpatient services and for short-term than for the long-term hospital stays" (Cafferata, 1985: 1094). One study of elderly patients living in five urban, low–income areas, noticed that those who had Medicare and Medicaid and used neighborhood centers as a regular source of care would use more ambulatory care than the average elderly patient (Wan, 1982: 96). Wan argued that the removal of financial barriers and "the innovative (outreach) approach of neighborhood centers in low–income areas had provided needed services to the poor and elderly individuals in low–income communities" (Wan, 1982: 96).

The Medicaid program, like the Medicare program, does not provide comprehensive health insurance coverage for its clients. Stuart, et al. explain that some of the causes for the statewide variation in Medicaid coverage are: 1) different eligibility criteria; 2) lack of uniform benefit packages, and 3) a variation in reimbursement rates across states (Stuart, et al., 1985: 95-96). Okada and Wan found that in five urban low–income areas:

> The Medicaid coverage of the poor ranged from 19% of the population in the Peninsula Charleston (SC) to 56% of the population in Roxbury (Boston, MA), in spite of the fact that the poverty level in these two areas was about equal (Okada and Wan, 1978: 339).

Aside from the regional variations noted above, Gortmaker found in a study of poor children in Flint, Michigan that "families with older children, more educated mothers, working mothers, and white families, tend not to be enrolled in Medicaid, independent of the eligibility criteria noted" (Gortmaker, 1981: 571), Davis and Rowland found that as a result of the various restrictions on Medicaid coverage, "about 60 percent of the poor are not covered by Medicaid" (Davis and Rowland, 1983: 157). Walden, et. al., mention that it is this same group of people who are ineligible for public insurance that are most likely to be uninsured since they also are least likely to have private insurance coverage as well (Walden, et al., 1985: 3).

Besides those who are most likely to be uninsured as a result of being ineligible for Medicaid, Walden, et al. found that the likelihood of being uncovered either part of the year or throughout the whole year was above the national average for young adults between nineteen and twenty-four, Hispanics and Blacks, the poor and other low–income groups (Walden, et al., 1985: 3). Mulstein suggests that one should add to the list of the uninsured the growing population of illegal aliens of which there is an estimated 3.5 to 6 million in the United States (with a large number in New York City and Los Angeles) who are uninsured and may avoid obtaining medical care because of the fear of detection (Mulstein, 1984: 217).

Although some of this group may be uninsured as a result of the gaps in coverage for those with public health insurance, some in fact may be uninsured because they are employed only part of the year; employed principally in the agriculture and forestry industries, personnel services, construction, retail industries; are self employed; work in firms with fewer than twenty-six employees; or work in firms with large low-wage forces (Mulstein, 1984: 216). Davis and Rowland as well as Aday, et al. found that the uninsured received considerably less care from physicians than the insured (Davis and Rowland, 1983: 160; Aday, et al., 1984: 86).

Davis and Rowland also note that there is a primary distinction between the categories of the uninsured, those who are always uninsured, and the sometimes uninsured.

> The always uninsured are individuals without Medicare, Medicaid or private insurance coverage for the entire year. . . The sometimes uninsured are those who were covered by public or private insurance part of the year but were uninsured the remainder of the year. The sometimes uninsured include the medically needy individuals who qualify for Medicaid coverage during periods of large medical expenses, but are otherwise uninsured (Davis and Rowland, 1983: 151–52).

On the other hand, those who are inadequately insured face the problem of only having coverage for some medical services; coverage only part of the year; coverage for inpatient hospital care, and not outpatient services; or coverage only for private, individually purchased coverage (Davis and Rowland, 1983: 151; Feder, et al., 1984: 546). Feder, et al. estimate that the figures for this group have fluctuated between 16.7 million in 1979 and 16.6 million in 1982 (Feder, et al., 1984: 546). One of the problems inherent in reporting the findings for the insured and the uninsured is that the uninsured may become insured after their savings run out. Thus while the statistics certainly suggest that there may be barriers to access for this group, the statistics may actually overestimate the lack of insurance coverage.

Methodological Issues

Although some multivariate models of utilization show factors such as regular source of care, insurance coverage, race, income, and residence to be less strongly associated with the use of medical care than expected, a multitude of studies do show that there is some relationship between these factors and utilization.

Mechanic hypothesizes that one possible reason for the discrepancies noted in studies of the use of medical care may be how the issues are "conceptualized, the nature of the measures used, the ways in which data are aggregated, and the manner in which analyses are performed" (Mechanic, 1979: 387). Mechanic further notes that in these studies proxy variables "for measuring morbidity are often correlated with various sociodemographic, attitudinal, and behavioral variables, and when introduced in multiple regression equations reduce the influence of such predictors" (Mechanic, 1979: 390). If this is true, this would suggest that there are multicollinearity problems in some of the multivariate models that may account for weak relationships between regular source of care, insurance, and access to medical care.

Kuder and Levitz examined the manner in which studies on the regular source of care and utilization of medical care are conducted. They noted that previous studies assumed either: that having a regular source of care *was important in determining* access to medical care because it led to an increased amount of medical care use by the patient (Model I), or that having or not having a usual source of care is *a consequence* of utilization and therefore is a function of the number of visits made to a physician (Model II) (Kuder and Levitz, 1985: 579-580). Rather than taking either assumption for granted, they tested the relationship between having a regular source of care and the use of medical care using cross-sectional data obtained from a household interview survey of residents of Washtenaw County, Michigan. They formulated three models to carry out this test. The first two models were based on the assumptions explained above, whereas the third model (Model III) assumed that "visiting the physician increases the likelihood of having a regular source *and* at the same time, that having a regular source also enhances access to a physician and thus increases use" (Kuder and Levitz, 1985: 580-83). They found that when one controls for other factors that Models II and

III had a smaller impact than Model I in determining the use of care (Kuder and Levitz, 1985: 594). They conclude:

> The results provide further evidence that the absence of linkages with a regular source is a significant barrier to ambulatory visits to the physicians and that population heterogeneity regarding such linkages is associated with variations in ambulatory care utilization (Kuder and Levitz, 1985: 594).

Aside from these issues surrounding the measurement of the regular source of care, Andersen, et al. present a host of other methodological problems that may hamper one's attempt to accurately study the relationship between the regular source of care, insurance coverage and realized access. Some of these issues include attempting to identify false negatives (i.e., "persons who did not report all their medical care experiences"), response biases due to survey nonresponse, under-reporting hospital payments for third party coverage (i.e., voluntary insurance, Medicare and Medicaid), and patients not accurately identifying major-medical coverage in their insurance policies (Andersen, et al., 1979: 122-127). In their 1970 national study of health care utilization and expenditures, Andersen, et al. report that despite these potential problems there were "few instances where the bias adjustments change the conclusions that would be drawn about the statistical significance of differences of health care experience between subgroups" (Andersen, et al., 1979: 126).

Cafferata explored some of the issues of measuring insurance coverage identified by Andersen, et al. She found that in a survey of the "most knowledgeable" elderly in the 1977 NMCES study, their knowledge of eleven health services programs was still rather low (Cafferata, 1984: 845). This knowledge tended to vary from a relatively high knowledge of the coverage of hospital services and surgery, slightly less knowledge about the coverage of dental and eye examinations, and less knowledge about the coverage of inpatient and outpatient mental health services (Cafferata, 1984: 845).

Cleary and Jette found, in a study of 1,026 persons over the age of eighteen, living in a three-county area containing approximately 50,000 people that people *under*-reporting outpatient visits were older (Avg. Age = 49.2 years) than those *over*-reporting these visits (Avg. Age = 38.4 years) (Cleary and Jette, 1984: 799).

Because older persons use more services these researchers conclude there is a tendency for high users of medical care to under-report the number of visits made to a physician (Cleary and Jette, 1984: 799).

Thus, if one accepts the argument that there are several potential sources of error in the multivariate studies, then one can conclude that some of the relationships concerning the role of regular source and insurance in determining access to medical care may actually be important but have not been adequately measured or conceptualized.

Summary

In summary, several multivariate studies of access to medical care have shown that health status variables, but not necessarily regular source of care and insurance coverage, are consistently important in determining medical utilization. However, other studies indicate that having a regular source of care plays an important role in determining the amount and type of utilization. There is also evidence that insurance coverage is important in determining access to medical care and that the amount of care received may vary by the extent of coverage. Some of the discrepant findings found in the literature may be due to measurement errors in the variables themselves or problems with the multivariate modeling of these relationships.

In the analyses that follow considerable attention will be given to considering the measurement of regular source of care and insurance coverage variables, understanding who has what kinds of coverage, and ultimately their levels of use and satisfaction — across a variety of national, state, and community data sets. Through a series of descriptive and multivariate analyses there will be an effort to explore and refine the policy, conceptual, and empirical utility of these care and coverage dimensions in understanding the organization and financing of the U.S. health care system and who is most likely to be affected by major policy changes in these areas.

Chapter 3
Description of Data Sets

CHRISTOPHER S. LYTTLE
LU ANN ADAY

FIVE DATA SETS were included in the analyses to address the probable impact of changes in the organization and financing of care on access to medical care — a 1982 national telephone survey, surveys of New York City and the poor in Arizona, and multi-site studies of a sample of eleven U.S. communities and five inner city areas in connection with evaluations of the Community Hospital Program (CHP) and Municipal Health Services Program (MHSP). Descriptions of the surveys and the comparability of data elements available from these studies are presented here.

Survey Design

1982 National Access Survey

In the spring and summer of 1982, Louis Harris and Associates conducted a national telephone interview survey of 3,000 families from a cross-sectional sample of the U.S. population. In addition, they oversampled approximately 1,800 families living in poverty. One interview was obtained with an adult in each family, a child (when present in the family) was also sampled, and an adult proxy interviewed about the sample child. This resulted in 6,610 individual (adult and child) interviews in 4,802 families. The overall response rate was 60 percent. A series of weights were applied to the data to adjust for 1) the fact of sampling only one adult and one child in each family; 2) the oversampling of families below poverty level; and 3) biases that might result from noncoverage due to households not having telephones; and 4) nonresponse. The study was funded by the Robert Wood Johnson Foundation (Princeton, NJ) and was intended to update the data available regarding the access impact in general and for the poor and disadvantaged in particular during a period of economically and politically motivated cutbacks in the availability of resources for medical care (Louis Harris and Associates, 1982a; Aday, et al., 1984).

Arizona Access Study of the Poor

The Flinn Foundation and the Robert Wood Johnson Foundation commissioned Louis Harris and Associates to conduct a telephone survey of the poor in Arizona during the late summer and early fall of 1982. The purpose of this study was to collect baseline information on the access of the Arizona poor prior to the implementation of the Arizona Health Care Cost Containment System (AHCCCS)—a program to bring Medicaid funds to the state for the first time and to develop and test a payment and delivery system for the state's poor and medically indigent. The survey was based on telephone interviews with adults living in areas of Arizona estimated to have a 20 percent or greater density of low-income families (excluding Indian reservations). Data were based on interviews with 2,500 adults and 1,155 children in families whose 1981 income was less than or equal to 200 percent of the AHCCCS program's indigency level. Once again, one adult and one child per family were chosen randomly for the study. Weights were assigned to reflect this sampling process. As with the New York study, final response rates do not appear in the final report for the study (Louis Harris and Associates, 1983). A report by the Flinn Foundation indicates that "completion rates among households meeting the income requirements were more than 90 percent. . ." (Flinn Foundation, 1985: 20). This completion rate estimate does not, however, adequately account for those who refused to participate at the time of initial income screening. In addition to the Harris and Flinn Foundation reports just cited, secondary analyses of the data have been conducted by the Center for Health Services Administration at Arizona State University (Kirkman-Liff, et al., 1982; Kirkman-Liff, 1984a; 1984b), and analyses comparing the 1982 baseline survey (included here) with a follow-up study in 1984 are also available (Flinn Foundation, 1985; Freeman and Kirkman-Liff, 1985).

Community Hospital Program (CHP) Evaluation

In the mid-1970s the Robert Wood Johnson Foundation launched a major program to improve the delivery of primary care through providing grant funds to over fifty community hospitals throughout the country to develop primary care-oriented group practices. The Center for Health Administration Studies, the University of Chicago, was awarded a grant to evaluate the impact of the groups on access to medical care in twelve of the fifty-three programs eventually funded by the foundation. (One group was dropped from the final study because it withdrew from the program, resulting in eleven communities being included in the final CHP access evaluation.) Two samples were drawn at each site for both the 1978-79 baseline (Time 1) and the follow-up (Time 2) some two years later. One sample was comprised of patients having visited the CHP site being evaluated, and the other consisted of individuals residing in the site's service area. The data presented here are predominantly from the area follow-up surveys in the eleven sites studied at that time (see descriptions in Table 3.1 Aday, et al., 1985).

Of all the studies included in these analyses, this is the only one in which the interviews were conducted on a face-to-face basis. One randomly selected adult and one randomly selected child were personally interviewed. The target was to complete 850 to 900 individual interviews in each site in each time period. The response rates for the follow-up community surveys varied from 72 percent to 90 percent and averaged 82 percent. The patient samples yielded response rates from 65 percent to 93 percent with an average of 81 percent. Weights were assigned as necessary to reflect differential sampling of households in some sites in the community samples as well as the number of individuals chosen from a family.

For most of the analyses presented here, the interviews from the follow-up community surveys in the eleven sites were combined. New weights were constructed for this purpose so that the contribution of each site to the weighted total was independent of any major differences *between* sites in their average weights. To accomplish this, an adjustment factor was assigned to make the

Table 3.1.   Selected Characteristics of the Community
Hospital Program Access Impact Evaluation
Sites.

CHP SITE	DESCRIPTION
01	Northeastern Central City of 138,000, Minority, Low Socio – economic Status
02	Southern Central City of 18,400, White, Low Socio – economic Status
03	Western Rural Area of 53,500, White, Lower Middle Class
04	North Central Suburb of 426,000, White, Middle Class
05	Southern Small Town of 22,900, White, Middle Class
06	North Central Mid-sized City of 72,600, White, Middle Class
07	Northeastern Rural Area of 22,300, White, Low Socio – economic Status
08	Southern Small Town of 41,600, White, Lower Middle Class
09	Western Suburb of 222,000, White, Middle Class (site excluded from study at Time 2)
10	Northeastern Suburb of 24,900, White, Middle Class
11	Southern Central City of 78,000, Black, Low Socio – economic Status
12	Western Central City of 629,000, Minority, Low Socio – economic Status

average case weight the same for each site. This means that the
relative contribution of a *site* is a function of its *actual sample size*
and the contribution of an individual *case* is a function of its
actual within-site weight. Because of the small weights required to
combine the patient list samples with the area samples, we have
elected not to use the list sample when computing community
estimates. When, as in Chapter 9, we combine CHP regular users
from the patient list and community samples, the analyses have
not been weighted.

Municipal Health Services Program (MHSP) Evaluation

Another major health care program initiative funded by the
Health Care Financing Administration (HCFA) and the Robert
Wood Johnson Foundation during the 1970s was the Municipal
Health Services Program (MHSP). This program was intended to
provide funds to the municipal hospital systems in five cities to
catalyze the development of primary care clinics that could
improve the delivery of care in the inner cities of Baltimore, Cincinnati, Milwaukee, St. Louis, and San Jose. In addition, HCFA

provided waivers for certain services not traditionally covered under Medicare for eligible patients who used the MHSP clinics.

The Center for Health Administration Studies conducted baseline and follow-up surveys in the service areas designated for each of the clinics in 1979 and 1982. A random digit dialing procedure was used to select phone numbers of potential respondents. To supplement the number of MHSP users in the sample, additional phone numbers of actual patients provided by the clinics were included in the bank of potential numbers. Households were screened at the time of the first telephone contact to see if anyone had used the facility. All households with members having visited an MHSP facility and a sample of households that had not were interviewed. Information was collected on all family members unless the family included more than six persons, in which case five members were randomly selected for the sample. This is the only study in this analysis where a single main respondent provides information on so many other family members. There is some evidence that reports on volume measures, such as number of visits to a physician, may decrease under this format (Andersen, et al., 1979). Approximately 1,000 families including 2,500 individuals were interviewed in each city. The completion rates in the follow-up surveys varied from 69 percent to 81 percent with an average of 73 percent. The sample was weighted to be representative of the noninstitutionalized community populations with home telephones. For the followup survey an additional weighting factor was applied to make the sample as representative as possible of the entire non-institutionalized population in the service areas, including those without telephones. As with the CHP study, for these analyses, data are included from the followup study only and combined across sites using weighting procedures comparable to those used for the CHP study (Fleming and Andersen, 1986).

New York City Access Study

In the spring and summer of 1982, Louis Harris and Associates conducted a telephone survey of a representative sample of New York City families, a city-wide oversample of low-income families with telephones and four special neighborhood samples drawn from one especially poor neighborhood in each of the Bronx, Manhattan, Brooklyn, and Queens areas. The study yielded a cross-section of 1,500 families in all five boroughs, 756 families whose 1981 income fell below 150 percent of the national poverty level, and a total of 1,513 or approximately 375 families from each of the neighborhood samples. As with the national study, interviews were obtained with one adult and, from an adult proxy, about one child (if present) in each family. There were 1,968 adults and children in the general cross-section sample, 1,041 in the low-income oversample, and 2,127 in the neighborhood samples. A final response rate is not reported in the final report on the study (Louis Harris and Associates, 1982b). Freeman and Lee, in a separate report on the survey do indicate, however, that "only about two out of three families contacted agreed to cooperate and be interviewed" (Freeman and Lee, 1984: 10), which could lead to biases in the data resulting from non-respondents being excluded.

The cross-section and low-income oversample were combined for the purpose of analysis and weighted as appropriate to integrate the low-income oversample. The four neighborhood samples were not included in these analyses since appropriate weights were not available to combine them with the other samples. As with the national study, weights were assigned to the adult and child records reflecting the number of adults and children in the family, to adjust for selecting only one adult and child. The New York study was funded by the Commonwealth Fund to provide input to inform their foundation's health program initiatives. The Fund worked closely with the Robert Wood Johnson Foundation and the Center for Health Administration Studies in an effort to maximize the comparability of the study with the 1982 national access survey. Further discussion of this study is available in Louis Harris and Associates (1982b), Mahoney (1982), and Freeman and Lee (1984).

Analytic Variables

All of the questionnaires used in the studies being analyzed here were based in part on earlier instruments developed by the Center for Health Administration Studies during the 1960s and 1970s. Because of this, the variables of interest are generally available and comparable in each of the data sets. All of the studies except for the CHP survey were conducted by telephone. The MHSP survey was designed to be a family level questionnaire, in which information was collected on up to five family members. Some items are not directly comparable due to these and other structural differences in the questionnaires. For example, in the CHP and MHSP studies data on reported medical conditions are gathered in the framework of an illness episode, whereas in the New York, Arizona, and 1982 national survey this information is gathered based on either conditions associated with the most recent physician visit, medical emergency, and/or hospital stay. Other incomparabilities between the data sets arise because some questions are not asked or are asked in a different fashion. The more significant of these are the lack of questions in MHSP about where people would go for care if they needed it even though they did not have a regular source; not obtaining income in a continuous form in the national, Arizona and New York studies; and the presence of symptom items only for the CHP and MHSP studies. Some detailed information is available in only one of the studies, such as selected preventative measures in the CHP study.

To enhance the basic comparability of the data elements, many of the key variables have been transformed to "reduced forms" which are as comparable across studies as possible. The algorithms for all reduced form variables eliminate, to the greatest extent possible, the minor variances in data elements across the data sets. This is shown in more detail for the Regular Source of Care and Insurance Variables in Tables 3.2 and 3.3. For example, in Table 3.2 it can be seen that for Arizona "County" and "Other" categories frequently had to be collapsed to create a category corresponding to the other studies. An important variance can be seen in Table 3.2 under "Reduced Form (1) Doctor's office or private clinic." HMOs have been coded into this category, but in CHP the reference is to "Group practices" and in MHSP there is no comparable category. In a few instances it remains important to remember that some items may not be strictly comparable across studies. Table 3.3 shows that for MHSP the categories "Prepaid group practice or HMO" and "Reduced rate clinic" were hand-coded out of the "Other" list, whereas in the other studies these were provided as explicit response categories to respondents at the time of the interview. The MHSP coding process represents a significant deviation from the procedure used in the other studies for two reasons: first, the respondent's judgment has been replaced by that of the coder; and, second, it makes the interpretation of the residual category "Other" more problematic. We do

Table 3.2. Sources for Reduced Form Categories—Regular Source of Care.

Category	STUDY				
	U.S.	Arizona	CHP	MHSP	NYC
1) Doctor's Office or Private Clinic	Doctor's Office or Private Clinic, HMO	Doctor's Office or Private Clinic, HMO	Doctor's Office or Private Clinic, Group Practice	Doctor's Office or Private Clinic	Doctor's Office or Private Clinic, HMO
2) Hospital OPD	Hospital OPD	County Hospital OPD, Other Hospital OPD, Unspecified Hospital	Hospital OPD	Hospital OPD	Hospital OPD
3) Hospital ER	Hospital ER	County Hospital ER, Other Hospital ER	Hospital ER	Hospital ER	Hospital ER
4) Other	Company or Union Clinic, School Clinic, Neighborhood or Government Sponsored Clinic, Other Place	Company or Union Clinic, Separate County Clinic or Primary Care Center, Unspecified Clinic, Some Other Kind of Clinic, Some Other Place	Company or School Clinic, Other Place	Neighborhood or Government Sponsored Clinic, Other Place	Company or Union Clinic, School and Unspecified Clinic, Neighborhood or Government Sponsored Clinic, Other Place
5) None	No Regular Source of Care	No Regular Source of Care	No Regular Source of Care	No Regular Source of Care	No Regular Source of Care

feel, however, that the construction of the reduced form variables with the aim of maximizing comparability should minimize the impact of any differences in the questions themselves across the studies on analytic outcomes.

Table 3.4 summarizes the major analytic variables to be used in the analyses. See Appendix A for a more complete description of the analytic variables.

Selection Variables refer to predisposing and enabling variables (such as age, sex, education, family size, etc.) of the behavioral model of health services utilization (Andersen, 1968). These categories of variables will be used to explain and, if necessary, modify the interpretation of the impact of the major organization

Table 3.3. Sources for Reduced Form Categories—Source of Insurance Coverage.

Category	STUDY				
	U.S.	Arizona	CHP	MHSP	NYC
1) Public Only	Medicare A, Medicare B, Medicaid or Public Aid	Medicare A, Medicare B, County Paid Medical Care	Medicare A, Medicare B, Medicaid or Public Aid, VA, CHAMPUS,	Medicare A, Medicare B, Medicaid/ Medi-CAL (DPA, Public Assistance), VA, CHAMPUS (coded out of "other")	Medicare A, Medicare B, Medicaid or Public Aid
2) Private Only	Through Work or Union, Through Some Other Group, Bought Directly, Prepaid Group Practice or HMO Other	Through Work or Union, Through Some Other Group, Bought Directly, Prepaid Group Practice or HMO Other	Through Work or Union, Through Some Other Group, Bought Directly, Prepaid Group Practice or HMO School Insurance Other	Through Work or Union, Through Some Other Group, Bought Directly, Prepaid Group Practice or HMO (coded out of "other") Remaining "others"	Through Work or Union, Through Some Other Group, Bought Directly, Prepaid Group Practice or HMO Other
3) Public and Private	Private and Public	Private and Public	Private and Public	Private and Public	Private and Public
4) None	Reduced Rate Clinic Residual Cases	Reduced Rate Clinic Residual Cases	Reduced Rate Clinic Residual Cases	Reduced Rate Clinic (coded out of "other") Residual Cases	Reduced Rate Clinic Residual Cases

and financing (means) variables on the access outcomes of interest.

The race and poverty level variables are of particular interest in this group of variables because they define the traditionally disadvantaged low-income and minority populations who are most apt to be affected by major health policy initiatives. Their potential and realized access profiles will be compared to the more advantaged higher income and majority white individuals.

The Need Variables represent both the subjective perception of the respondent as to state of health (perceived health, worry)

Table 3.4.   Index to Analytic Variables.

I. **SELECTION VARIABLES**

A. PREDISPOSING

A.1.   Age (continuous)
A.2.   Age (categorical)
A.3.   Sex
A.4.   Education of adult respondent
A.5.   Employment status of adult respondent
A.6.   Occupation of adult respondent
A.7.   Education of main wage earner
A.8.   Employment status of main wage earner
A.9.   Occupation of main wage earner
A.10.   Minority status
A.11.   Hispanic origin
A.12.   Race—reduced form
A.13.   Family size

B. ENABLING

B.1.   Family income (continuous)
B.2.   Family income (categorical)
B.3.   Family income—reduced form (high, medium, low)
B.4.   Poverty level

II. **NEED VARIABLES**

A.1.   Self-perceived health
A.2.   Worry
A.3.   Bed days in last year
A.4.   Non-hospital days in bed during last year
A.5.   Other disability days in last year
A.6.   Total disability days in last year
A.7.   Symptoms
A.8.   Number of symptoms
A.9.   Symptom severity index

III. **SYSTEM VARIABLES**

A. RESIDENCE

A.1.   Location (FIPS code)
A.2.   Location—reduced form (region)
A.3.   Residence (central city, SMSA, etc.)
A.4.   Residence—reduced form
A.5.   Length of residence in city, neighborhood

B. AREA RESOURCE FILE (ARF)

B.1.   Physician supply (MDs per 1000 population)
B.2.   Per capita income

IV. **MEANS VARIABLES**

A. REGULAR SOURCE

A.1.   Is there a regular source of care?
A.2.   Description of regular source of care
A.3.   Is it an HMO?
A.4.   Regular source of care—reduced form
A.5.   If no "regular place", is there a "might go" place?
A.6.   Description of place "might go"
A.7.   Is it an HMO?

B. INSURANCE COVERAGE

B.1.   Any insurance coverage?
B.2.   County paid medical care?
B.3.   Health insurance through work or union?
B.4.   Health insurance through some other group?
B.5.   Health insurance bought directly by yourself?
B.6.   Medicare A?
B.7.   Medicare B?
B.8.   Medicaid or Public Aid?
B.9.   Prepaid group practice or HMO?
B.10.   Another clinic or center with reduced rates?
B.11.   Any other place?
B.12.   Veteran's Administration?
B.13.   CHAMPUS?
B.14.   School insurance?
B.15.   Insurance coverage—reduced form

V. **ACTUAL ACCESS VARIABLES**

A. CONVENIENCE

A.1.   Waiting time

B. UTILIZATION—contact and Volume

B.1.   M.D. contact in last year (Y/N)
B.2.   House calls by a doctor or doctor's assistant

Table 3.4.   Index to Analytic Variables. *(Continued)*

B.3.	Visits to a doctor's office or private practice	B.21.	Visit mix (ER-OPD vs. other)
B.4.	Visits to a group practice		**C. SATISFACTION**
B.5.	Visits to a county clinic		
B.6.	Visits to a non-county clinic	C.1.	Satisfaction with office waiting time
B.7.	Visits to a company or union clinic	C.2.	Satisfaction with out-of-pocket cost
B.8.	Visits to a school clinic	C.3.	Satisfaction overall
B.9.	Visits to a neighborhood or government clinic		**D. TYPE OF SERVICE**
B.10.	Visits to a hospital outpatient clinic	D.1.	Preventative measures (within year)
B.11.	Visits as a hospital inpatient		Had a blood pressure reading
B.12.	Visits to a hospital emergency room		Had a pap smear for cancer
B.13.	Visits to a county emergency room		Had a breast examination by a doctor
B.14.	Other (non-county) emergency room visits	D.2.	Use-Disability ratio
B.15.	Visits to any other place		**E. EXPENDITURES**
B.16.	Sum of physician visits		
B.17.	Hospitalizations in last year (Y/N)	E.1.	Hospital inpatient
B.18.	Number of admissions	E.2.	Ambulatory OPD and ER
B.19.	Number of nights	E.3.	Other ambulatory physician
B.20.	Visit mix (inpatient vs. outpatient)	E.4.	All other

and more objective measures of health needs (number of days in bed, conditions precipitating various actions, symptoms experienced).

The System Variables in Table 3.4 refer to aggregate county data descriptive of the health care system and the population in the areas studied. These secondary data were obtained from the Area Resource File (ARF) (U.S. Department of Commerce, 1984) and linked to the records of individuals at the county level by using Federal Information Processing Standard (FIPS) codes. The ARF is a collection of data compiled from different sources. The variables considered in this study came primarily from the American Medical Association Physician Master File, the County-Level Hospital File from the American Hospital Association Annual Survey, the 1980 Census of Population, and the 1975-1980 Local Area Personal Income (U.S. Department of Commerce, 1984: 119). Many variables from the ARF were considered and tested for inclusion in our analyses; however, ultimately, only two were used — a physician supply variable and per capita income variable.

The Means Variables are the major analytic variables of interest here. These variables reflect the organizational and financing dimensions of care discussed in Chapter 1. These dimensions are operationalized through descriptors of the regular source of care and insurance coverage, reported by respondents. Another analytic variable is a typology resulting from the cross-classification of the regular source of care and insurance coverage variables. This variable is used to look at the impact of the interaction and combination of financial and organizational factors on access to health care.

The Actual Access Variables are the primary outcome variables in the Behavioral Model and represent a number of different dimensions of access to care. Convenience is measured by the time spent waiting at the source of care prior to seeing a physician. Utilization refers to the services (physician visits and hospitalizations) actually consumed. Satisfaction is measured for the most recent contact with the health care delivery system. Type of service primarily refers to categories of preventive health care procedures as well as the ratio of visits to days of disability experienced. Finally, expenditures for selected inpatient and outpatient services are also examined.

Summary

Five data sets were included in the analyses to address the probable impact of changes in the organization and financing of care on access to medical care — a 1982 national telephone survey, surveys of New York City and the poor in Arizona, and multi-site studies of a sample of eleven U.S. communities and five inner city areas in connection with evaluations of the CHP and MHSP. These studies collected data between early 1981 and late 1982, with most of the interviews conducted in 1982. Because earlier questionnaires developed by the Center for Health Administration Studies were the basis for the design of many of the questions asked in these studies, there is a consistency in the availability of data elements as well as a considerable degree of comparability among data elements in the various studies.

Chapter 4
Analytic Plan

RONALD M. ANDERSEN

THIS CHAPTER describes the analytic plan for the empirical analyses that will be used to address the research questions posed in this study. The major questions are of two types:

1) What are the major differences in sources and financing of medical care for different segments of the U.S. population?

2) What impact do differences in sources and financing of care have on access to medical care measured by convenience, volume, and types of services received, use relative to need, as well as consumer satisfaction with these services?

Answers to these questions will be used to suggest how current and proposed changes in organization and finance might affect the access to and use of medical services.

Dimensions of the Analytic Plan

The two dimensions of the analytic plan are displayed in Figure 4.1. The rows of the figure represent the types of analysis to be performed beginning with the simplest and most descriptive (row 1) and concluding with the most complex, multivariate and special analyses (row 7). The columns show the various data sets used in the analysis, beginning with the national data (column 1) and following with data from other studies representing various sectors of the U.S. population (columns 2 through 5). The cells formed by the rows and columns provide a framework for describ-

Figure 4.1. Analytic Plan

Types of Analysis	Data Sets				
	National (1)	Arizona Low Income (2)	New York City (3)	Community Hospital Program (CHP) (4)	Municipal Health Services Program (MHSP) (5)
(1) Regular Source	X	X	X	X	X
(2) Insurance Coverage	X	X	X	X	X
(3) Regular Source and Insurance Coverage for Subgroups	X				
(4) Health Care Need According to Regular Source and Insurance Coverage	X	X	X	X	X
(5) Outcome According to Regular Source and Insurance Coverage	X				
(6) Multivariate Analyses	X				
(7) Special Sample Analyses	X	X	X	X	X

X = Data set employed in this analysis.

ing the particular kinds of analysis planned for each data set. An "X" in a particular cell means the analysis was performed using the corresponding data set.

Types of Analysis (Rows of Figure 4.1)

1. Regular Source

This analysis will focus on regular source of care as a prime enabling variable. As indicated in Chapter 2, regular source may impact on the care people receive in a variety of ways. These include: (a) whether or not people get care at all; (b) the mix of services they receive (e.g., inpatient vs. outpatient); (c) whether primary services (prevention) or secondary (treatment) services are emphasized; (d) the degree of continuity and integration there is in planning and treating a patient during an episode of illness; (e) the appropriateness of the treatment; (f) the cost of care; and (g) consumer satisfaction with the care received. Because of the numerous ways regular source of care can influence a patient's experience in obtaining medical care, an additional assumption is that ultimately the overall health and well-being of the patient may be affected by these experiences — although this assumption will not be tested directly in this analysis. In addition to exploring where people usually go for care we will: (1) for those who do *not* have a regular source, look at whether they have some place they *might* go if they needed medical attention; and (2) make comparisons of those for whom not having a regular source of care is voluntary, or their own choice, with those for whom it is not really a choice.

2. Insurance Coverage

The other important enabling variable in this analysis is the kind of health insurance people have. The financing of medical care has been shown to be at least as important, if not more important, an influence on care received than regular source. All of the outcomes thought to be affected by regular source may also be influenced by insurance coverage including getting care at all, whether or not having a regular source is voluntary, the mix of services received, emphasis on prevention or treatment, continuity, quality, cost, and consumer satisfaction. Indeed, financing also directly influences what the regular source will be.

3. Regular Source and Insurance Coverage for Subgroups

A major part of the analysis will focus on what impact regular source of care, insurance coverage, and the combination of the two have on access to medical care for various subgroups in the U.S. population. Of special interest will be the source of care and insurance coverage for different income and ethnic groups. Other population subgroups to be studied include those defined by sex, age, and place and region of residence. The basic analysis of who has what types of care and coverage will be addressed in Chapter 5.

4. Health Care Need According to Regular Source and Insurance Coverage

As we contemplate policy changes that impact on consumers' regular source of care and insurance coverage, an important question is, "Are there different levels of illness and health care needs for various groups who have different patterns of care and coverage?" Answers to this question are needed to give us some better idea of what might happen to costs and use of service as people shift from one source to another (e.g., private doctors' offices to hospital OPDs) or change their insurance coverage (e.g., Medicaid to no coverage). A consideration of how medical need differs for different groups will be reported in Chapter 6.

5. Outcome According to Regular Source and Insurance Coverage

Row 5 signifies the shift in the analysis from questions of who has various kinds of care and insurance coverage to those about outcome or what difference these organization and financing dimensions make in terms of access outcomes such as the convenience of care, volume and mix of service, prevention or curative emphasis, and consumer satisfaction with care. These access outcome analyses will be the focus of Chapter 7.

6. Multivariate Analyses

The next stage of the analysis (Chapter 8) will be a multivariate, multistage effort to model who has what kind of care and insurance and the subsequent impact of this organizational and financial access on utilization. The advantage of this approach is that a number of factors can be simultaneously considered. It also helps to visualize and quantify the dynamics of the selection and impact of a source of care and insurance on the ultimate subjective and objective outcomes of patient access, outlined in our framework in Chapter 1 (Figure 1.1).

7. Special Sample Analyses

Finally, the unique characteristics of the special samples (Arizona, NYC, Community Hospital Program (CHP) and Municipal Health Services Program (MHSP)) allow us to address other important access questions. In Chapter 9 we will use multivariate analyses to consider (1) What is the access to care of low–income people living in areas with different Medicaid coverage (NYC and Arizona)? (2) Does access differ among Hispanics of Mexican and Puerto Rican origin and Blacks living in different communities (Arizona, NYC, and selected CHP and MHSP samples)? (3) How does access differ for people using innovative forms of ambulatory care (CHP and MHSP) compared to those using more traditional sources? and (4) Do health care expenditures vary among people using traditional versus innovative sources of care (MHSP) regularly?

Data Sets (Columns of Figure 4.1)

1. National

The national study data represented by column 1 in Figure 4.1 is the primary data set for the analysis. Most of the analyses will utilize this national data set since it does provide information on the country as a whole. The operational definitions of the study variables were developed using variables available in the national study as the main point of reference.

The other data sets representing the low–income population of Arizona, New York City, communities from the Community Hospital Program and communities from the Municipal Health Services Program will be used more selectively. The purposes of these selective analyses will be to: (1) confirm findings from the national study using multiple data sets; (2) elaborate some investigations where the additional data sets have richer, more detailed information; and (3) address questions uniquely suited to these additional study populations. Some special questions that the various data sets are especially well-suited to address are discussed below, and will be emphasized, especially, in the final analytic chapter (Chapter 9) on special access issues and problems.

2. Arizona Low-Income

These data were collected prior to the Arizona Health Care Cost Containment experiment. At that time Arizona had no Medicaid program and the eligible poor were treated at county facilities. Thus, we have the opportunity to compare regular sources of care and access for the poor people without Medicaid to sources of care and access of the poor with traditional Medicaid coverage in the other studies. The Arizona study also allows us to look at a special Hispanic group—those living in Arizona, largely of Mexican heritage.

3. New York City

This sample provides the opportunity to look at the effects of a quite liberal state Medicaid program on access for the poor. Also, New York City supports an extensive Public Hospital System. This sample also provides a special view of a significant Hispanic group of largely Puerto Rican origin and a large urban black population.

4. Community Hospital Program (CHP)

The CHP samples provide information on rural, suburban, and large central city populations, as well as communities which are predominantly Black or Hispanic. The CHP surveys allow us to look at the impact of a special variant of community hospital sponsored care, which attempted to incorporate elements of private medical group organization and primary care emphasis. We will compare this program with other types of ambulatory care arrangements found in our samples. The CHP data set also includes a symptoms-checklist and illness episode questions which enable a more detailed look than most of our data sets at the appropriate use of services relative to need (Aday, et al., 1985).

5. Municipal Health Services Program (MHSP)

The MHSP samples provide a detailed access picture of central city areas across the country. Of special interest is the MHSP effort to provide public sponsorship of primary care centers in the neighborhood away from the campuses of the public hospital. This study also provides information on what happens under a more comprehensive Medicare program, covering items such as drugs and dental care, for example. We feel it will be informative to compare access outcomes for people in these programs with the variety of alternative combinations of regular source of care and health insurance coverage found in our other data sets. The MHSP samples have considerable information on communities of central city Hispanics and Blacks, as well as the majority White population. The MHSP data set also offers detailed expenditure data to examine some of the trade-offs between access and the costs of medical care for people with different sources of regular care.

Summary

This chapter has outlined the analysis plan for the study. We will first construct measures of regular source of care and insurance coverage. We will then describe the status of the country with respect to regular source and insurance coverage using the above measures. The next part of the analysis will examine the regular care and insurance coverage of various subgroups in the country focusing on income and ethnic groups. Next, we will address the relative need for care of people who go to different sources. We will then turn to the question of the impact of organization and financing on outcome for patients measured in terms of convenience, the nature and appropriateness of services received, and consumer satisfaction. The final part of the analysis will attempt, using multivariate analysis, to model the process of obtaining a regular source of care and insurance coverage and the special access problems and outcomes for people with different sources of care and coverage.

The above questions will be addressed using the national data set first. The other data sets in the secondary analysis will be used to confirm and elaborate the national findings and to address special questions for which various of these data sets are uniquely suited.

Chapter 5
Sources and Financing of Medical Care

RONALD M. ANDERSEN,
CHRISTOPHER S. LYTTLE
LLEWELLYN J. CORNELIUS

THIS CHAPTER answers the first major study question outlined in the introduction of the analytic plan in Chapter 4: What are the major differences in sources and financing of medical care for different segments of the U.S. population? The specific issues addressed in this chapter are: 1) What are people's regular sources of medical care? 2) What kinds of insurance coverage do they have? and 3) What combinations of regular care and insurance coverage are most frequently found in the United States? We will then explore the characteristics of people with different kinds of care and insurance coverage.

Characteristics of U.S. Population and Subsamples

As background for the analyses to follow, we will first consider some population characteristics of the various samples included in the study. Some understanding of the distribution of relevant predisposing, enabling, and need variables within these samples is helpful in understanding people's choice of a regular source of care and type of insurance coverage.

Table 5.1 shows that young children and the elderly make up a sizable proportion of each sample (16 percent or more). The Arizona low-income sample includes the most young children (12 percent). The New York City (NYC) sample has the fewest under six years of age (8 percent). The Community Hospital Program (CHP) and Municipal Health Services Program (MHSP) samples include the same proportion of elderly as the national sample (11 percent), while Arizona has more elderly (14 percent) and NYC has less (8 percent).

The minority distributions are very different from sample to sample (Table 5.1). All subsamples except Arizona have more Blacks than the national sample (11 percent). NYC leads with 21.6 percent of the sample being Black. The Hispanic distribution ranges widely from 7 percent in the CHP sample to 59 percent of the Arizona low-income sample. One-fourth of the NYC sample is Hispanic.

Education levels are highest in the national and NYC samples where 81 and 74 percent report completing high school. About two-thirds of the CHP and MHSP samples finished high school, while less than one-half of the Arizona sample did so.

Turning to enabling characteristics, the subsamples generally have proportionately more persons below the poverty level than the national sample (14 percent). By definition the Arizona low-income sample are *all* below poverty level. All the special samples are more urban and less rural than the national sample. Again, by definition, the MHSP and NYC samples are totally central city sites. There are suburban and rural communities included in the CHP sample and in Arizona but *on average* these samples are more urban than the nation.

Table 5.1 reveals a similar proportion reporting fair or poor health in the national, CHP, MHSP, and NYC samples (15 to 19 percent). The proportion in Arizona (32 percent) was considerably higher. There was somewhat less variation in the average number of disability days per person per year, ranging from a low of 15 in the national, CHP, and NYC samples to a high of 23 in Arizona.

Regular Sources of Care

Table 5.2 shows the distribution of regular sources of care in the national study as well as in each of the special surveys. The categories of regular care chosen for these analyses represent the modal types used in this country. Earlier studies also suggest that these types result in different patterns of care and costs of services. Private offices and clinics, which includes group practices and HMOs, are the most common type. While there is great heterogeneity within type, qualities attributed to the private office include an emphasis on primary and continuous care, a de-emphasis on specialized and inpatient care, and, possibly, lower costs. The hospital sources, both outpatient departments (OPDs) and emergency rooms (ERs), are associated with more specialized, less continuous services. They are also associated with higher overall costs due to the higher overhead of providing care in the hospital and the tendency to use the more complex and costly technology readily available in the hospital setting. We separate the OPD from the ER because patients in the former are more likely to have prior appointments, records available when they come for care, and some familiarity with the providers treating them. "Other" is a heterogeneous category including school and industrial facilities as well as free clinics, neighborhood health centers, maternal and child health centers, and other publicly sponsored programs that respondents might consider as a regular source of care. Finally, there is the category of persons who can identify no particular place they go for medical care or for advice about their health. This group has been a prime target of new organization and financing efforts because it is usually assumed to be underserved or inappropriately served.

Table 5.2 shows that almost three-quarters of the people in the national survey and CHP samples named a private office or clinic as their regular source of care. Recall that the CHP sample represents a combination of urban, suburban, and rural communities. The MHSP and NYC samples reported fewer private office sources although this category was still the most frequently mentioned source. Both of these latter samples represent urban central city populations. Finally, the Arizona sample reported the fewest private doctor sources (38 percent). This is a low–income sample in a state without Medicaid at the time of the survey. Consequently, we are viewing a group less likely to have personal resources or private insurance to purchase private physician services. They also lack publicly sponsored Medicaid that would allow some of them to receive private physician services that could be paid for by public insurance.

Hospital OPDs are the second most frequently reported regular sources of care in all samples (Table 5.2). The county hospitals used by the low–income population in Arizona explain why so many low–income people in that state (29 percent) report a hospital OPD as a regular source of care. New York City with the largest urban area in the United States and a huge public hospital system has 12 percent reporting an OPD as the regular source of care. Hospital OPDs are also named as regular sources by 12 percent of the sample in the MHSP study. MHSP samples are all from large urban areas. Proportionately fewer named an OPD in the national (7 percent) and CHP (7 percent) samples.

Hospital ERs are named less frequently than OPDs as regular sources of care (Table 5.2). Still, in the MHSP sample 5 percent did so. Even in the national sample the 2 percent naming ERs represent close to five million people in this country.

The "Other" category is named frequently enough to be policy-relevant in every sample. There is a great range in the proportions of "others"—from 5 percent in the CHP and national samples to 15 percent in the Arizona sample. The county facilities described by the low-income population in Arizona as government clinics may explain why the latter percent is this large.

Eleven percent of the U.S. population reported no regular source of care. Similar proportions were found in the CHP (13 percent) and NYC (12 percent) samples. The proportions without regular care in the Arizona and MHSP samples were larger (15 percent each). Both of these samples represent low-income populations which are generally less likely to have a regular source of care. Thus, in all samples, but particularly in the low-income ones, we find sizable proportions of the population who have not established regular ties with the health care system.

There are varying degrees of knowledge of and association with sources of care. Even those persons who do not admit to having a regular source of care may have a place in mind they would go in an emergency. In all but the MHSP study those without a regular source of care were asked where they might go (Table 5.3).

In the national sample about one-half of those without a regular source reported a particular doctor's office or clinic where they would go if they needed medical care. About one-third had nowhere in mind to go. The remainder of the people without a regular source were spread about equally among the remaining sources of care. Proportionately more name an ER as a place they would go (5 percent) than had named it as a regular source (2 percent). This is not surprising since emergency services are often represented as "backup" services. In fact, one might have expected the 5 percent to be higher, with more of those having no place they "regularly go" to have named an ER as where they "might go" if they needed care.

The results in Table 5.3 for Arizona differ considerably from the national sample. Only a quarter of those without a regular source report a private office as a place they might go. About one-fifth of them report a hospital OPD and around one-tenth an ER as a place they might go. Fully two in five have nowhere in mind to go. The greater dependence on hospital facilities or no source in Arizona might again reflect the low-income composition of this sample.

The CHP and NYC responses by persons without a regular source of care (Table 5.3) are also different from the national sample. Over one-half the people in both these samples could not name a place they might go. Further, fewer of them mentioned a private office as a place they might go than in the national sample.

In sum, one-quarter to one-half of the people without a regular source of care named a private office where they might go in the various samples. One-third to one-half did not mention any source. In general, a higher proportion of those without a regular source of care mentioned a hospital facility as a place they might go than the proportion of all people who reported having a hospital facility as a regular source would go initially. Still, hospital facilities are not mentioned as frequently as doctors' offices as places those without a regular source would go, except for the low-income population in Arizona.

As indicated in earlier chapters, many positive outcomes are commonly attributed to having a regular source of care. These include propensity to seek care when needed, compliance with medical regimen, continuity of care, prevention of acute episodes, and monitoring of chronic conditions. Despite such positive attributes some people do not want a regular source of care. Table 5.4 shows the reasons people give for not having a regular source in the three studies (national, Arizona, and CHP) where the question was asked. The responses are divided into those we call "voluntary" — suggesting people freely choose not to have a regular source — and "involuntary" — suggesting some barrier inhibits them from establishing a regular source.

Two-thirds or more of the reasons given in all of the studies indicate a voluntary decision to not have a regular source. By far the most common reason given (about one-half of all reasons) is simply that they feel they do not need a regular source or seldom go to a physician. Behind this general reason is the sense that they do not feel sick enough, or sufficiently vulnerable to illness, to spend the time and money to establish a regular source. Another group of voluntary reasons amounting to more than one-tenth of the reasons given in each study suggest that people do get care more or less regularly, but may not identify with a particular doctor or place. These people report they use specialists, have "no particular doctor", or go to various ERs or clinics. Some of the voluntary reasons (5 to 8 percent) imply displeasure with medical care—people do not like doctors or report poor care from the past. Finally, a few people are voluntarily without a regular source because they usually see a relative or friend for their health care needs.

The reasons we labelled as "involuntary" were given less frequently, ranging from 29 percent in the national study and CHP to 34 percent in Arizona. In Arizona (a low-income sample) the most common reason (19 percent) was "can't afford a regular source." A fairly common response in all sites (9 to 12 percent) is "have moved recently." It suggests a transitory period after a move which puts people "out of reach" of their former regular source; possibly, they have not yet gathered information, had the time, or felt the need to establish themselves with a new regular source. Another reason given (accounting for as much as 7 percent in the national and CHP samples) is that the old doctor is unavailable—probably because of moving, retiring, dying, or limiting practice. Finally, a small percentage in each site claimed "they did not know any doctor."

In sum, Table 5.4 indicates that the majority of people without a regular source of care think they do not need one. If indeed a policy maker believes the benefits of regular source care merit pursuing this group—either a healthy dose of health education or a considerable reduction in the perceived price (time, effort, or money) of establishing a relationship with a regular provider may be needed. A minority mention some barrier to obtaining a regular source. Of those who "moved recently" some will presumably right the situation in due course. Those who believe they can't afford a regular source represent a group for whom the "price" of a regular source may also need to be reduced if the goal of increasing regular linkages with the health care system is to be achieved.

Insurance Coverage

The insurance coverage for the U.S. population and selected subgroups is given in Table 5.5. Persons sixty-five and over are separated from those under sixty-five because all older people are assumed to be covered by Medicare and thus have some insurance. Coverage is divided into public sources, private sources, and no insurance. People can also be covered by more than one of these major types of insurance.

Public sources are divided into Medicare, Medicaid, and other public sources. The latter includes CHAMPUS (insurance for dependents of armed forces personnel) and Veterans Administration services for former armed forces personnel.

Private insurance includes health insurance purchased from Blue Cross/Blue Shield; investor-owned insurance companies such as Travelers, Prudential, and Aetna; as well as coverage through HMOs, preferred provider organizations, and other innovative forms of health care financing through private sources. Private insurance is separated in Table 5.5 into group insurance obtained through employer groups and other group memberships, such as the Grange, professional organizations or organizations of retired persons, and individual insurance purchased directly by individuals or families from insurance agents.

Those who report that they receive care "free" or at reduced rates from a particular health facility may receive services through public hospitals, community health centers, or "free care clinics." They are viewed as having more financial subsidies for medical care than people without any insurance. However, those reporting free care are generally considered to have a more transitory and less comprehensive means of obtaining care than those with some formal type of insurance coverage.

The final category of "none" is a residual group. In Table 5.5 it includes people with no public or private insurance or free care.

The most common form of coverage for those under sixty-five is group insurance, held by well over one-half of the people in all samples except Arizona where the proportion is 42 percent. The second most common coverage varies from sample to sample. It is individually purchased insurance in the national and NYC samples. Medicaid or county coverage ranks second for the MHSP sample of inner city residents and the Arizona low-income sample. Medicaid and individually purchased insurance are each held by almost one-tenth of the people in the CHP sample, representing diverse communities. Medicare covers a small percentage of persons under sixty-five in each sample including the disabled, blind, and persons on kidney dialysis. Free or reduced-rate care is reported by a substantial proportion of the low-income population in Arizona (17 percent) and 8 percent of the national and NYC samples. Finally, almost one-third of the Arizona sample reported no insurance and no source of reduced rate care. A smaller but still policy-relevant percentage of the other samples (10 to 14 percent) reported having no kind of health care coverage.

Table 5.5 shows that many elderly have coverage supplementary to Medicare. Almost one-third to over one-half of the various samples of people sixty-five or over report group insurance coverage. Such coverage could be retained through their previous employment or obtained through groups such as the National Association of Retired Persons. Others obtain additional coverage by purchasing policies through Blue Cross or other insurance companies (27 to 45 percent). Medicaid also provides supplementary coverage for those who cannot pay the Medicare deductibles or coinsurance or exhaust their Medicare benefits and personal resources. Seventeen percent of the elderly in the national and NYC samples and smaller proportions in the other samples report Medicaid coverage. Few elderly report obtaining free or reduced rate care.

Table 5.6 shows the combinations of health insurance held by those under sixty-five and the elderly. Seventy percent or more of the non-elderly in all of the samples except the Arizona low-income sample hold private insurance only. In the latter low-income sample only 37 percent have private insurance only. However, more of the Arizona sample (20 percent) report public insurance only (the county coverage that preceded Medicaid in Arizona). "Public and Private" coverage for those under sixty-five is sometimes reported by people who had private insurance which was not adequate to cover their medical expenses. They are eligible for Medicaid because of their limited income or by "spending down" their personal resources for medical services until they qualify for Medicaid. The percentage reporting public and private coverage in the various samples ranged from 2 to 6 percent. The proportion under sixty-five who have no insurance or whose only relief from medical expenses is care at a free or reduced rate clinic is 37 percent in Arizona but considerably less in the other samples (11 to 14 percent).

Table 5.6 shows that 77 percent of those sixty-five and over report multiple public and private coverage in the national sample. In all of the other samples more than one-half of the elderly report public and private coverage except Arizona, where multiple coverage is still reported by 45 percent. Multiple coverage generally implies something different for the elderly than for the under sixty-five population, who tend to be a low-income group eligible for Medicaid all or part of the year. In contrast, the elderly with both public and private coverage tend to be the better-off group, who can afford to supplement their Medicare with additional Blue Cross or other private health insurance.

There has been a recent spurt in HMO enrollment across the nation that has significant implications for the overall financing and organization of health services in the country. Since most of the interviewing covers 1982 or earlier in the studies discussed here, current coverage would be considerably higher. Seven percent of the U.S. population reported HMO membership (not shown in a table). The reported HMO coverage varies considerably among the other samples — from a low of 1 percent in the CHP sample to as much as 13 percent in the NYC sample.

The kind of insurance coverage one has may play a major role in determining whether the person has a regular source of care and what that source might be. Table 5.7 shows what types of regular care people have for each type of insurance coverage.

A majority of people in most insurance categories, including those with no insurance, report a private doctor as their regular source of care (Table 5.7). The proportions range from a high of 78 percent of those under sixty-five who have private insurance only to a low of 55 percent of those under sixty-five who have no insurance. A hospital OPD or ER or other clinic is frequently mentioned as a source of care for people under 65 with public insurance only (36 percent). Those without insurance are most likely to have no regular source of care (21.6 percent).

Lack of any insurance coverage is generally viewed as a major barrier to appropriate medical services and a serious threat to the financial stability of an individual or family, should catastrophic illness occur. Still some people choose not to purchase health insurance, gambling that they will not incur medical expenses they cannot manage or that someone else will foot the bill should they become ill. None of our studies provide direct information on why people do not have health insurance. However, given the costs of insurance that would cover substantial hospital and physician charges, low-income people are less likely to have the option to purchase health insurance on their own. In the absence of insurance they are likely either to be inhibited from seeking care or dependent on charity care. Table 5.8 shows the income status of people with and without health insurance. Fifty-six and 67 percent of those without insurance in the national sample and the CHP subsample were at or below the poverty level (defined here as 150 percent of the Bureau of Labor Statistics poverty level). Thus, we might conclude that more than one-half of the uninsured have little choice in the matter, given financial realities. Others without insurance above the poverty level may have the resources to purchase some health insurance, but for many of these a significant financial barrier probably remains.

People with Various Sources of Care and Coverage

In this section we will use the national sample to examine the social and demographic characteristics of people with different kinds of regular sources, insurance coverage, and combinations of these. The particular characteristics examined are shown in Table 5.9. They were chosen because they represent groups that have traditionally been thought to be disadvantaged in terms of medical care access and/or have been targeted for special medical care programs.

Table 5.9 indicates that the people who go to private physicians' offices are less likely to be below the poverty level and Black than those having other sources of care. People who regularly use the hospital OPD include disproportionate numbers of poor, Blacks, elderly, the less-educated, and both central city and rural farm residents. Regular ER users look like OPD users with the following notable exceptions: they include fewer females, children, elderly, and rural farm residents. The other clinic population is similar to the outpatient population in most characteristics. Those without a regular source of care actually appear to be better off financially and include fewer minorities than those who use hospitals but include slightly more of the traditionally disadvantaged groups than those with a private doctor; and are more likely to be living in the central city. They are less likely to be female, children, or elderly than those with a private doctor.

Table 5.10 shows the characteristics of people under sixty-five according to their insurance coverage. Persons with public insurance only include disproportionate numbers of most disadvantaged groups. Of particular note is the low income and education level of this group and the relatively large proportions who are Black and children and live in central cities. Such characteristics reflect the largely Medicaid population found in the public only group under sixty-five. Southern residents tend to be *underrepresented* in this group, reflecting the more restrictive Medicaid programs in this region.

The private only insurance group has the highest level of education and income and the lowest proportion of minorities and people living in central cities of any insurance group.

The public and private insurance group tends to be less disadvantaged than the public only group but more disadvantaged than the private only. Remember this is a group that may be eligible for Medicaid sometimes (when the main earner is not working or the family has high medical expenses) and not eligible at other times. Thirty percent of this group is below the poverty level compared to over 60 percent of the public only group, but only 8 percent of the private only group.

The uninsured people under sixty-five, who make up 10 percent of the non-elderly, are between those who have both public and private insurance with regard to their disadvantaged status. They are more like those with private coverage with respect to age, sex, proportion Black, and proportion living in the South. They have less education and income than the private group but considerably more education and income than the public only group. A unique characteristic of the uninsured is that they represent the highest proportion of Hispanics of any insurance group.

Table 5.11 compares the characteristics of people sixty-five and over who have public insurance only (Medicare or Medicare plus Medicaid) with those who have both public insurance and a supplementary private policy. On almost all counts those with supplementary insurance are a more advantaged group. They have more income and education and are less likely to be minority. The elderly with more resources purchase additional insurance to cover Medicare coinsurance and deductibles, to pay for services Medicare does not include such as drugs, and to provide for catastrophic medical expenses after Medicare benefits are exhausted. The poorer elderly must more often rely on Medicaid or charity programs to cover these contingencies.

Table 5.12 allows us to look at the kinds of people who have various combinations of regular sources of care and insurance coverage. The majority (66 percent) of the population have a private doctor and some private health insurance. This group has higher income and education levels than any other group in the typology. They represent the group we would expect to have the fewest access problems.

Persons without any regular source of care or insurance represent the other extreme of the categories in Table 5.12. They are a small portion of the population (2 percent) but are expected to have the most problems in getting medical care. They are less-educated, have relatively lower incomes and are more likely to be Hispanic and live in central cities than the population as a whole.

People with other combinations of regular source and insurance described in Table 5.12 might be expected to have access problems of magnitudes somewhere between those of the extreme groups discussed above. The three categories with public insurance only have some common characteristics. They include large numbers of elderly and persons with low education and income levels. Those with public insurance and a private doctor are particularly likely to be female. Those with public insurance who use hospital facilities or other clinics are more likely to be Black and central city residents. Finally, publicly insured individuals with no regular source of care are a very small proportion of the total population and include disproportionate numbers of the elderly.

Persons with some private insurance who either use hospital facilities or have no regular source are among the largest categories in the typology (11 and 8 percent) after the private doctor-private insurance group. Both of these groups include large proportions of males. Those using hospital facilities are more likely to be central city residents than people in other private insurance categories.

The remaining categories in Table 5.12 not previously discussed include people without insurance that go to a private doctor or use a hospital facility. They are similar to those without insurance who have no regular source; relatively large proportions are Hispanic. While all groups without a regular source have income and education levels lower than people with insurance and a private doctor, they are better off than the groups that have public insurance only. While economic barriers are one reason people may not have a regular source, the most important reason reported earlier in the chapter (Table 5.4) was that they did not need one.

Summary

In this chapter we have explored the regular sources of medical care people have and the nature of their health insurance coverage. We considered reasons for not having a regular source and the relationship between health insurance coverage and poverty. Finally, we examined the social and economic characteristics of people with different sources of care and insurance coverage. We next turn to the illnesses and health needs of these people.

Table 5.1. Population Characteristics of the U.S. Population and Selected Subgroups.

CHARACTERISTICS	U.S.	ARIZONA Low Income	CHP	MHSP	NYC
Predisposing					
Female	52%	58%	52%	54%	56%
Under 6	9	12	10	11	8
65 and Over	11	14	11	11	8
Black	11	9	15	13	21
Hispanic	8	59	7	14	25
Less than High School	19	60	33	35	26
Enabling					
Family Income <$7,500	13	72	19	21	20
Below 1.0 Poverty	14	100	18	25	-
Central City	29	48	36	100	100
Rural Farm	4	-	1	-	-
South	34	-	39	20	-
Need					
Fair or Poor Health	15	32	16	17	19
Total Non-Hospital Disability Days (Mean Days)	15	23	15	19	15
Table n	6610	3655	5691	13271	3009

Table 5.2. Regular Source of Care for the U.S. Population and Selected Subgroups.

REGULAR SOURCE	U.S.	ARIZONA Low Income	CHP	MHSP	NYC
Private Office/Clinic	74%	38%	73%	59%	65%
Hospital OPD	7	29	7	12	12
Hospital ER	2	2	3	5	4
Other	5	15	5	9	7
Company/Union Clinic	1	2	–	–	3
School Clinic	1	–	*	*	*
Government Clinic	3	9	4	9	3
Unspecified Clinic	–	3	–	–	–
Some Other Place	1	*	1	*	1
No Regular Source of Care	11	15	13	15	12
Total	100%	100%	100%	100%	100%
Table n	6561	3628	5675	13251	2935

---

* = less than 0.5 percent.

Table 5.3. Where People without a Regular Source of Care Might Go if They Needed Care for the U.S. Population and Selected Subgroups.

"MIGHT GO" SOURCE	U.S.	ARIZONA Low Income	CHP	MHSP	NYC
Private Office/Clinic	51%	24%	34%	-	37%
Hospital OPD	6	19	4	-	5
Hospital ER	5	9	5	-	3
Other	6	7	2	-	4
Company/Union Clinic	1	1	*	-	2
School Clinic	1	-	*	-	1
Government Clinic	4	3	1	-	2
Unspecified Clinic	-	3	-	-	-
Some Other Place	*	*	1	-	*
No Place They Might Go	33	40	55	-	51
Total	100%	100%	100%	-	100%
Table n	682	511	750	-	358

* = less than 0.5 percent.

Table 5.4.   Reasons for Not Having a Regular Source of
Care for the U.S. Population and Selected
Subgroups.

REASONS	U.S.	ARIZONA Low Income	CHP
Voluntary	71%	65%	71%
Don't Need One	50	48	49
Seldom Go to MD	2	2	3
No Particular MD	7	6	4
Care from Army, VA	2	*	2
Use Specialists	2	*	2
Clinic, Emergency Room	2	4	4
Don't Like MDs	4	3	5
Previous Care Poor	1	2	3
Relative, Friend	1	*	1
Involuntary	29%	34%	29%
Moved Recently	12	9	11
Old MD Not Available	7	3	7
Can't Afford Regular MD	7	19	4
Don't Know any MD	2	2	1
Other	1	1	6
Number of Responses	814	630	863

* = less than 0.5 percent.

Table 5.5.   Insurance Coverage for the U.S. Population and Selected Subgroups by Age.

INSURANCE COVERAGE	U.S.	ARIZONA Low Income	CHP	MHSP	NYC
		Percent Under 65 with . . .			
Public					
Medicare	2%	5%	1%	2%	4%
Medicaid/County	5	22	9	15	12
Other Public	-	-	3	1	-
Private					
Group	80	42	72	69	70
Self	26	16	8	7	22
No Insurance					
Free Care	8	17	*	*	8
None	10	30	11	13	14
Table n	5564	2946	5100	11836	2608
		Percent 65 and Over with . . .			
Public					
Medicare	100%	100%	100%	100%	100%
Medicaid/County	17	14	9	7	17
Other Public	-	-.	2	1	-
Private					
Group	55	45	30	38	45
Self	45	30	27	29	40
No Insurance					
Free Care	5	6	*	*	3
None	-	-	-	-	-
Table n	1046	709	591	1435	366

---

* = less than 0.5 percent.

Table 5.6.   Combinations of Public and Private
Insurance Coverage for the U.S. Population
and Selected Subgroups by Age.

INSURANCE COVERAGE	U.S.	ARIZONA Low Income	CHP	MHSP	NYC
		Percent Under 65 with . . .			
Public Only	3%	20%	10%	14%	10%
Private Only	83	37	77	71	71
Public & Private	4	6	2	3	5
No Insurance	11	37	11	13	14
Total	100%	100%	100%	100%	100%
Table n	5538	2887	5087	11836	2608
		Percent 65 and Over with . . .			
Public Only	23%	55%	45%	36%	35%
Public & Private	77	45	55	64	65
Total	100%	100%	100%	100%	100%
Table n	1046	709	591	1435	366

Table 5.7. Regular Source of Care by Insurance Coverage for the U.S. Population by Age.

REGULAR SOURCE OF CARE	INSURANCE COVERAGE				
	Public Only	Private Only	Public & Private	No Insurance	Total
Percent Under 65 with . . .					
Private Office/ Clinic	57%	78%	70%	55%	75%
Hospital OPD	19	5	9	12	7
Hospital ER	5	1	1	3	2
Other	12	5	9	8	5
No Regular Source of Care	7	10	11	21	11
Total	100%	100%	100%	100%	100%
Table n	267	4138	281	831	5517
Percent 65 and Over with . . .					
Private Office/ Clinic	70%		77%		75%
Hospital OPD	12		11		11
Hospital ER	*		2		1
Other	7		5		5
No Regular Source of Care	11		6		7
Total	100%		100%		100%
Table n	326		707		1033

---

* = less than 0.5 percent.

Table 5.8. Poverty Level Status of the Insured and
Uninsured Populations Below 65 for the
U.S. Population and CHP Subsample.

| POVERTY LEVEL | INSURANCE COVERAGE | |
	YES	NO

U.S. POPULATION

Equal to or Below 1.5 Poverty	19%	56%
Above 1.5 Poverty	81	44
Total	100%	100%
Table n	4714	824

CHP POPULATION

Equal to or Below 1.5 Poverty	24%	67%
Above 1.5 Poverty	76	33
Total	100%	100%
Table n	4527	560

Table 5.9.   Characteristics of People According to Their Regular Source of Care for the U.S. Population.

CHARACTERISTICS	REGULAR SOURCE					
	Private Office/ Clinic	Hospital OPD	Hospital ER	Other	No Regular Source of Care	Total
Predisposing						
Female	54%	51%	36%	51%	41%	52%
Under 6	10	8	i	8	3	9
65 and Over	11	17	10	10	7	11
Black	8	20	20	19	13	11
Hispanic	8	9	11	11	9	8
Less than High School	18	22	27	24	21	19
Enabling						
Below 1.0 Poverty	12	23	21	23	17	14
Central City	26	41	37	37	32	29
Rural Farm	4	7	2	4	3	4
South	34	32	33	29	37	34
Table n	4779	523	130	407	722	6561
Percent of Population	74%	7%	2%	5%	11%	100%

Table 5.10. Characteristics of People According to Their Insurance Coverage for the U.S. Population (Under 65).

CHARACTERISTICS	INSURANCE COVERAGE				
	Public Only	Private Only	Public & Private	No Insurance	Total
Predisposing					
Female	60%	51%	49%	52%	51%
Under 6	17	9	9	11	10
Black	28	10	24	13	11
Hispanic	11	8	10	14	9
Less than High School	46	14	37	32	17
Enabling					
Below 1.0 Poverty	62	8	30	39	14
Central City	46	26	37	36	28
Rural Farm	3	4	1	6	4
South	23	34	33	38	35
Table n	268	4165	281	824	5538
Percent of Population	3%	83%	4%	10%	100%

Table 5.11. Characteristics of People According to Their Insurance Coverage for the U.S. Population (65 and Over).

CHARACTERISTICS	INSURANCE COVERAGE		
	Public Only	Public & Private	Total
Predisposing			
Female	61%	58%	59%
Black	11	7	7
Hispanic	9	2	4
Less than High School	46	30	34
Enabling			
Below 1.0 Poverty	28	12	16
Central City	29	31	31
Rural Farm	4	4	4
South	33	31	31
Table n	330	716	1046
Percent of Population	23%	77%	100%

Table 5.12.   Characteristics of People According to the Typology of Consumers' Care for the U.S. Population.

TYPOLOGY

CHARACTERISTICS	Public Insurance			Some Private Insurance			No Insurance			Total
	Pvt. M.D.	Hosp. ER/OPD	None	Pvt. M.D.	Hosp. ER/OPD	None	Pvt. M.D.	Hosp. ER/OPD	None	
Predisposing										
Female	61%	58%	55%	54%	47%	38%	55%	54%	47%	52%
Under 6	8	9	3	9	6	2	13	11	6	9
65 and Over	59	37	66	10	13	6	-	-	-	11
Black	11	36	12	8	18	13	10	19	11	11
Hispanic	9	14	13	7	10	8	16	11	14	8
Less than High School	45	52	43	15	19	18	33	29	31	19
Enabling										
Below 1.0 Poverty	41	53	35	8	15	10	36	42	40	14
Central City	33	45	32	25	37	29	30	43	43	29
Rural Farm	4	4	1	4	5	3	7	6	4	4
South	31	27	13	34	30	40	41	39	32	34
Table n	401	137	55	3922	727	477	439	192	187	6537
Percent of Population	3%	1%	*	66%	11%	8%	5%	2%	2%	100%

* = less than 0.5 percent.

Chapter 6
Health Care Needs

MEEI-SHIA CHEN

LLEWELLYN J. CORNELIUS

As MENTIONED previously, one of the important issues in formulating health policy is determining whether people with different types of care and coverage also have different needs for medical care. The desire to highlight the importance of health care needs in the selection of a particular source of care or insurance coverage is premised on the assumption of the importance that equitable factors, such as the actual need for care, as well as enabling factors, such as having a regular source of care and insurance, play in the actual use of services (Andersen, 1968). This chapter will describe the patterns of health needs that exist for individuals with different types of care and coverage across the five studies, as well as set the stage for measuring the possible effects these and other factors have on access to medical care in the chapters that follow.

A variety of measures of need will be presented in this chapter: patients' perceptions of their health level, based on self-reports of whether their health is excellent, good, fair, or poor and the extent to which they worry about their health; behavioral indications of whether they may have had to limit their usual activity because of illness, based on a count of the days respondents state that they were restricted in their ordinary activity (disability days); the number of symptoms they reported having in the year, as a signal of acute morbidity; and finally an evaluation of the severity of these symptoms by a panel of physicians as a provider-based indicator of medical needs. We shall look at all these measures to determine any potential variance in need patterns for people with different types of care and coverage.

Perceived Health

Perceived health has been found to be an important correlate of health services utilization. This measure of need is based on the respondents' evaluation of their health to be excellent, good, fair, or poor. Table 6.1 summarizes the proportion of people with fair or poor perceived health by age for people with different types of or no regular source of care. The general pattern for both those under sixty-five and sixty-five and over across different studies shows that hospital outpatient department (OPD) users had the highest proportions reporting fair or poor health and those who had no regular source of care the lowest. When one compares the users of hospital emergency rooms (ERs) with either the users of private offices or clinics, or other types of clinics, which include company/union clinics or government clinics, hospital ER users seemed to be somewhat "sicker" than these other groups.

A closer look at Table 6.1 reveals that some groups sixty-five or over had higher proportions with fair or poor health than expected. For example, 91 percent of hospital ER users sixty-five or over in Arizona and 57 percent of the elderly in New York City (NYC) who did not have regular sources of care had fair or poor health—much higher than the general pattern. However, these estimates are based on a small number of respondents in the respective subgroups.

Not only does one find a pattern when looking at perceived health by respondents' regular source of care, but also by their type of insurance coverage (Table 6.2). For example, for those under sixty-five the proportions with fair or poor health were highest among those who had public insurance only or had both public and private insurance. This suggests that public insurance programs such as Medicaid or Medicare serve people with greater needs. On the other hand, people who only had private insurance had the best health status, as indicated by a much lower proportion with fair or poor health in this group. Those without insurance coverage were not as healthy as the individuals with private insurance only but were healthier than those having some types of public insurance. Among those sixty-five or over, those who had both public and private insurance perceived themselves to be healthier than those who only had public insurance (principally Medicare).

Worry

The amount of worry associated with the respondent's health was based on a scale of "a great deal", "some", "hardly any", or "none". It is another respondent-based evaluation of health. This measure was only used in the Community Hospital Program (CHP) and Municipal Hospital Services Program (MHSP) studies (Tables 6.3 and 6.4). A significantly smaller proportion of people under sixty-five without a regular source of care in both the CHP and MHSP studies (15 and 18 percent) worried about their health, compared to those with some place they routinely went to for care.

A greater proportion (34 and 32 percent for CHP and MHSP) of regular hospital OPD users under sixty-five had a great deal or some worry about their health than regular users of private doctors, hospital ERs, and other clinics. A lower percentage of regular hospital ER users (21 and 27 percent) worried about their health when compared to the users of private doctors and other sources of care. Therefore, regular ER users, although having a lower level of perceived health than the latter two groups, worried less about their health. This is probably a function of the larger proportion of younger regular ER users who tended to worry less overall. We found (data not shown) that a much higher percentage of regular ER users (37 and 47 percent in the CHP and MHSP samples), compared with a lower proportion of private doctor users (21 and 28 percent in the CHP and MHSP samples) and other clinic users (24 and 28 percent in the CHP and MHSP samples), are eighteen through thirty-four years of age. The pattern of the amount of worry by regular source of care for those sixty-five and over was similar to those under sixty-five.

Table 6.4 once again summarizes a familiar pattern: individuals under sixty-five who had some type of public insurance had greater needs as measured by the degree to which they worried about their health, than those who had no insurance or had only private insurance coverage. For those sixty-five and over, those with public insurance (effectively Medicare) only in the CHP study had a greater amount of worry about their health than those with public and supplementary private insurance coverage.

Disability Days

Total disability days is another important measure of need. It includes estimates of non-hospitalized bed days and other days respondents may have had to cut down on the things they usually do. Reported in Tables 6.5 and 6.6 are estimates of the mean number of total disability days for subgroups with or without various regular sources of care or insurance for the five studies. Overall, regular OPD users had, in general, higher disability days (21 to 26) and individuals without a regular source of care had the lowest (6 to 13) total disability days (bottom of Table 6.5). In the Arizona study the low-income individuals who regularly used private doctors had about the same number of disability days (27) as hospital OPD users (26). Regular ER users in the national study had much higher numbers of disability days (34), mostly due to the extremely high average number of disability days (186) for those sixty-five and over. There was not a consistent pattern of disability days across the studies for the users of private doctors, hospital ERs, or other clinics. In the national, Arizona, and CHP studies, those who regularly used "other" sources for care had fewer disability days than those who regularly used hospital ERs or private doctors for care. On the other hand, hospital ER users seemed to fare better in the MHSP study and worse in the national study, than the users of private doctors or other clinics.

Table 6.6 indicates that public insurance programs, as mentioned earlier, were serving people with greater needs, i.e., people under sixty-five who had some form of public insurance had a greater average number of disability days. Among those under sixty-five, people who had private insurance only or were uninsured tended to have lower numbers of disability days. However, the health status of the individuals who only had private insurance were not much better off than those without insurance, if total disability days, rather than perceived health, or amount of worry about health, is used as the measure of need.

We have shown that those sixty-five and over with public insurance only had poorer perceived health than those who had supplementary private insurance coverage across five studies.

However, only in the CHP and NYC studies did the former group have a greater number of disability days than the latter.

Symptoms

Another self-assessed measure of need is the number of symptoms respondents reported to have experienced in the past year based on a checklist of fifteen symptoms incorporated in the CHP and MHSP questionnaires. Tables 6.7 and 6.8 summarize the mean number of symptoms reported for selected subgroups.

Overall, regular hospital OPD users had the greatest number of symptoms while those without a regular source of care had the smallest number of symptoms in both the CHP and MHSP studies. As is expected from previous discussions, hospital OPD users had the worst health status and those who did not have a regular source of care had the best health, according to this indicator. In the CHP study, regular hospital ER or other clinic users had somewhat fewer symptoms than those using private offices/clinics regularly. However, these three groups were similar in their number of symptoms in the MHSP study. In Table 6.8 we see that those under sixty-five with public insurance reported higher number of symptoms than those with private insurance or those without insurance. For those sixty-five and over, there is little difference between those with public insurance only and those with both public and private coverage.

Mean Severity Index of Symptoms

A final measure of need that will be considered in this chapter is a mean severity index of the symptoms reported above. A panel of physicians evaluated the severity of the types of symptoms reported by the patient which may be used to provide some further validation of the patients' evaluations of their health needs. Each doctor was asked to estimate, based on training and experience, how many people out of one hundred manifesting a certain symptom should see a doctor for it. The ratings for each symptom were obtained for each of five patient age groups: 1-5, 6-15, 16-44, 45-65, and 65 and over. An individual's severity index was obtained by summing the estimated ratings for all of the symptoms reported (Aday, et al., 1980).

Tables 6.9 and 6.10 report the mean severity of symptoms for the CHP and MHSP studies according to one's regular source of care and type of insurance coverage. Table 6.9 indicates that the users of hospital OPDs had more severe symptoms than other users, whereas those with no regular source of care had the least severe symptoms, according to the panel of physicians. Likewise, Table 6.10 indicates that those with some form of public insurance had the more severe symptoms and those with private insurance or no insurance had the least severe symptoms.

The findings on this and the previous patient-reported indicators of health status suggest that those with public insurance or users of hospital OPDs not only tend to be sicker than those with other types of care or coverage, but may have more severe illnesses, thus reflecting a greater overall need for care.

Special "Needs" Issues

Considering that those with private insurance or users of private doctors are in better health than those with public insurance or users of hospital OPDs, it is possible that the combination of these care and coverage factors may result in variant patterns of health as well. So far we have described the need of subgroups in terms of their regular source of care and insurance coverage *separately*. Given the possible influence that a combination of care and coverage may have on access it is also useful to examine the needs of people simultaneously based on the organization and financing dimensions of care. A typology was constructed to look at these possible interactions by combining various regular sources of care and insurance coverage. Using perceived health as an example, Table 6.11 shows the combined effects of care and coverage: the proportions with fair or poor perceived health were much higher among regular hospital OPD users who had some form of public coverage but much lower among those who had no regular source of care but did have some form of private insurance. The table also reveals that those with public insurance, regardless of their sources of care, had poorer perceived health than those who had either private insurance or no insurance.

The patterns of need across the measures of perceived health, amounts of worry, disability days, number of symptoms, and the mean severity index indicate that those who had private insurance or no insurance or had no regular source of care reported the best health on all the measures, whereas those who had public insurance or used hospital OPDs regularly had poorer perceived health than the other groups.

One may conclude from these findings that those without a regular source of care or insurance coverage, should not be of concern to health professionals since they have better health. However, as mentioned previously in Chapter 5 people without a regular source of care may include those who freely choose not to have a regular source (voluntary reasons) as well as those who are not able to have a regular source of care because of some type of barriers (involuntary reasons). Further, the no insurance group includes those who are at or below 150 percent of the poverty level and those who have incomes greater than 150 percent of the poverty level. The former are less likely to have the option to purchase health insurance because of financial barriers. The health patterns of these groups may be very different. Tables 6.12 and 6.13 show the percent with fair or poor health and mean disability days for these groups. Table 6.12 indicates clearly that, in the national, Arizona, and CHP studies, those who did not have a regular source of care for involuntary reasons were much more likely to have fair or poor perceived health than those who voluntarily chose not to have a regular source. Although the "voluntary" group had better health than those *with* a regular source, the "involuntary" group was not necessarily better off. For total disability days, there were no significant differences between the "involuntary" and "voluntary" groups in the national and CHP studies. But the former still averaged more disability days in the Arizona study.

Table 6.13 shows that among those under sixty-five who do not have insurance in the national and CHP studies the poor and the near poor had much poorer perceived health and greater total disability days than those above the poverty level. In effect, the former group had even a greater proportion with fair or poor health and more mean disability days than those *with* insurance coverage.

The analysis of people without regular source of care or insurance coverage demonstrates that, to better understand the needs of these people, health policy makers need to make finer distinctions as to (1) whether or not the individual has a choice in having a regular source of care, and (2) whether the uninsured are poor or not.

Summary

Based on the analyses of the variety of measures of need for those with particular types of care and coverage reported in this chapter, the following patterns emerge: (1) regular OPD users were sicker than those who either use a private doctor as their regular source of care or who did not have a regular source of care; 2) people who were enrolled in public insurance programs had greater needs than those who had only private insurance coverage or were uninsured; 3) these patterns are in general similar for those under and over sixty-five years of age; 4) the sample of the low–income population in Arizona were "sicker" than those in other studies across all the measures of health care needs examined.

These findings pose the question of whether those who select a particular type of care or coverage are having their needs adequately met. This question will be explored further in the chapters that follow.

Table 6.1 Percent with Fair or Poor Health According to Regular Source of Care for the U.S. Population and Selected Subgroups by Age.

REGULAR SOURCE	PERCENT WITH FAIR OR POOR HEALTH				
	U.S.	ARIZONA Low Income	CHP	MHSP	NYC
Under 65					
Private Office/Clinic	11%	28%	12%	13%	14%
Hospital OPD	22	35	24	20	30
Hospital ER	19	31	17	17	19
Other	15	26	14	14	20
No Regular Source	10	22	9	11	12
Total	12	29	13	14	16
Table n	5512	2907	5079	11799	2530
65 and Over					
Private Office/Clinic	38%	51%	43%	36%	44%
Hospital OPD	38	67	55	54	55
Hospital ER	(61)	(91)	(49)	54	(33)
Other	25	71	(61)	41	54
No Regular Source	26	25	19	25	57
Total	37	54	42	37	47
Table n	1029	684	585	1433	358
Total					
Private Office/Clinic	14%	33%	16%	16%	17%
Hospital OPD	24	39	27	23	33
Hospital ER	23	40	19	18	20
Other	16	29	19	16	23
No Regular Source	11	22	10	12	16
Total	15	32	16	17	19
Table n	6541	3591	5664	13232	2923#

( ) = based on 25 or fewer unweighted cases.
Subgroup n's do not sum to total due to missing values on age.

Table 6.2   Percent with Fair or Poor Health According
             to Insurance Coverage for the U.S.
             Population and Selected Subgroups by Age.

INSURANCE COVERAGE	PERCENT WITH FAIR OR POOR HEALTH				
	U.S.	ARIZONA Low Income	CHP	MHSP	NYC
Under 65					
Public Only	39%	37%	28%	25%	28%
Private Only	9	24	10	11	11
Public and Private	27	33	32	32	30
No Insurance	20	30	16	14	22
Total	12	29	13	14	16
Table n	5517	2869	5081	11815	2562
65 and Over					
Public Only	49%	59%	51%	41%	61%
Public and Private	33	49	35	35	40
Total	37	54	42	37	47
Table n	1042	690	586	1434	364

Table 6.3 Percent for Whom Health Caused a Great Deal or Some Worry According to Regular Source of Care for CHP and MHSP by Age.

REGULAR SOURCE	PERCENT HEALTH CAUSED WORRY	
	CHP	MHSP
Under 65		
Private Office/Clinic	30%	31%
Hospital OPD	34	32
Hospital ER	21	27
Other	28	31
No Regular Source	15	18
Total	28	29
Table n	5075	11795
65 and Over		
Private Office/Clinic	48%	44%
Hospital OPD	(59)	51
Hospital ER	(53)	(29)
Other	(57)	39
No Regular Source	(28)	32
Total	47	43
Table n	590	1427
Total		
Private Office/Clinic	32%	32%
Hospital OPD	37	33
Hospital ER	22	27
Other	31	31
No Regular Source	16	19
Total	30	30
Table n	5665	13222

( ) = based on 25 or fewer unweighted cases.

Table 6.4   Percent for Whom Health Caused a Great Deal or Some Worry According to Insurance Coverage for CHP and MHSP by Age.

INSURANCE COVERAGE	PERCENT HEALTH CAUSED WORRY	
	CHP	MHSP
Under 65		
Public Only	36%	39%
Private Only	27	26
Public and Private	46	48
No Insurance	23	25
Total	28	29
Table n	5077	11811
65 and Over		
Public Only	54%	44%
Public and Private	42	43
Total	47	43
Table n	591	1428

Table 6.5   Mean Number of Total Non-Hospital
Disability Days According to Regular Source
of Care for the U.S. Population and Selected
Subgroups by Age.

REGULAR SOURCE	MEAN DISABILITY DAYS				
	U.S.	ARIZONA Low Income	CHP	MHSP	NYC
Under 65					
Private Office/Clinic	12	20	14	16	13
Hospital OPD	17	21	18	20	20
Hospital ER	19	19	13	13	21
Other	12	14	8	14	13
No Regular Source	6	12	6	9	7
Total	12	18	13	15	14
Table n	5318	2898	4927	11417	2537
65 and Over					
Private Office/Clinic	36	53	34	45	32
Hospital OPD	60	67	50	85	20
Hospital ER	(186)	(45)	(75)	50	(5)
Other	17	64	(46)	48	49
No Regular Source	34	23	8	31	(34)
Total	40	53	33	48	31
Table n	905	678	574	1401	359
Total					
Private Office/Clinic	15	27	17	20	15
Hospital OPD	23	26	21	26	23
Hospital ER	34	22	16	14	21
Other	12	17	12	17	15
No Regular Source	8	13	6	11	9
Total	15	23	15	19	15
Table n	6223	3576	5501	12818	2931

( ) = based on 25 or fewer unweighted cases.

Table 6.6   Mean Number of Total Non-Hospital
Disability Days According to Insurance
Coverage for the U.S. Population and
Selected Subgroups by Age.

INSURANCE COVERAGE	MEAN DISABILITY DAYS				
	U.S.	ARIZONA Low Income	CHP	MHSP	NYC
Under 65					
Public Only	43	30	25	23	25
Private Only	10	14	11	13	11
Public and Private	37	26	40	49	23
No Insurance	12	15	10	11	14
Total	12	18	13	15	14
Table n	5322	2860	4929	11432	2569
65 and Over					
Public Only	33	53	39	43	46
Public and Private	41	54	28	50	23
Total	39	53	33	48	31
Table n	915	682	575	1402	365

Table 6.7 Mean Number of Symptoms Reported According to Regular Source of Care for CHP and MHSP by Age.

REGULAR SOURCE	MEAN SYMPTOMS	
	CHP	MHSP
Under 65		
Private Office/Clinic	1.67	1.09
Hospital OPD	2.25	1.27
Hospital ER	1.36	1.14
Other	1.22	1.08
No Regular Source	1.14	0.85
Total	1.60	1.08
Table n	4965	11817
65 and Over		
Private Office/Clinic	2.63	2.02
Hospital OPD	3.20	2.56
Hospital ER	(2.76)	2.05
Other	(4.38)	2.37
No Regular Source	1.37	1.41
Total	2.60	2.05
Table n	590	1434
Total		
Private Office/Clinic	1.78	1.21
Hospital OPD	2.36	1.39
Hospital ER	1.45	1.18
Other	1.55	1.19
No Regular Source	1.16	0.89
Total	1.71	1.18
Table n	5555	13251

( ) = based on 25 or fewer unweighted cases.

Table 6.8   Mean Number of Symptoms Reported According to Insurance Coverage for CHP and MHSP by Age.

INSURANCE COVERAGE	MEAN SYMPTOMS	
	CHP	MHSP
Under 65		
Public Only	2.27	1.45
Private Only	1.48	1.00
Public and Private	2.99	2.11
No Insurance	1.65	0.91
Total	1.60	1.07
Table n	4967	11836
65 and Over		
Public Only	2.56	2.12
Public and Private	2.63	2.00
Total	2.60	2.05
Table n	591	1435

Table 6.9   Mean Severity Index of Symptoms Reported
According to Regular Source of Care for
CHP and MHSP by Age.

REGULAR SOURCE	MEAN SEVERITY OF SYMPTOMS	
	CHP	MHSP
Under 65		
Private Office/Clinic	0.98	0.64
Hospital OPD	1.33	0.77
Hospital ER	0.79	0.66
Other	0.74	0.65
No Regular Source	0.65	0.48
Total	0.94	0.63
Table n	4965	11541
65 and Over		
Private Office/Clinic	1.64	1.26
Hospital OPD	1.99	1.62
Hospital ER	(1.74)	1.28
Other	(2.84)	1.48
No Regular Source	(0.85)	0.90
Total	1.63	1.28
Table n	590	1434
Total		
Private Office/Clinic	1.06	0.72
Hospital OPD	1.41	0.85
Hospital ER	0.85	0.68
Other	0.96	0.72
No Regular Source	0.66	0.51
Total	1.02	0.70
Table n	5555	12975

( ) = based on 25 or fewer unweighted cases.

Table 6.10   Mean Severity Index of Symptoms Reported
             According to Insurance Coverage for CHP
             and MHSP by Age.

INSURANCE COVERAGE	MEAN SEVERITY OF SYMPTOMS	
	CHP	MHSP
Under 65		
Public Only	1.38	0.88
Private Only	0.86	0.58
Public and Private	1.77	1.29
No Insurance	0.96	0.53
Total	0.94	0.63
Table n	4967	11559
65 and Over		
Public Only	1.61	1.34
Public and Private	1.64	1.24
Total	1.63	1.28
Table n	591	1435

Table 6.11   Percent with Fair or Poor Health According to Typology for the U.S. Population and Selected Subgroups.

TYPOLOGY	PERCENT WITH FAIR OR POOR HEALTH				
	U.S.	ARIZONA Low Income	CHP	MHSP	NYC
Private Doctor					
Public Insurance	47%	49%	38%	30%	42%
Private Insurance	12	28	12	14	14
No Insurance	15	31	18	15	17
Hospital OPD					
Public Insurance	42	48	37	38	47
Private Insurance	19	32	21	18	24
No Insurance	35	37	(28)	18	36
Hospital ER					
Public Insurance	(54)	(67)	(27)	30	(38)
Private Insurance	(17)	(36)	(16)	17	(10)
No Insurance	(37)	(25)	(20)	(12)	(31)
Other Source					
Public Insurance	(42)	34	(29)	22	50
Private Insurance	13	30	(15)	14	18
No Insurance	(16)	24	(8)	14	(13)
No Regular Source					
Public Insurance	(27)	(21)	(24)	18	40
Private Insurance	8	22	8	11	12
No Insurance	23	24	(12)	12	20
Table n	6530	3533	5631	13232	2913

( ) = based on 25 or fewer unweighted cases.

Table 6.12   Percent with Fair or Poor Health and Mean Total Non-Hospital Disability Days by Choice and Lack of a Regular Source of Care for the U.S. Population and Selected Subsamples.

	U.S.			ARIZONA			CHP		
	Has Regular Source	Has No Regular Source		Has Regular Source	Has No Regular Source		Has Regular Source	Has No Regular Source	
		Involuntary	Voluntary		Involuntary	Voluntary		Involuntary	Voluntary
Percent with Fair or Poor Health									
Less than 65	12%	15%	8%	30%	25%	20%	13%	12%	7%
65 and Over	38	(42)	18	58	(54)	14	36	(30)	(15)
Total	15	17	9	34	27	19	17	14	8
Table n	5856	237	453	3085	190	314	4867	257	474
Total Non-Hospital Disability Days (Mean Days)									
Less than 65	13	8	5	19	16	9	14	7	5
65 and Over	40	9	(45)	57	(41)	15	36	(7)	9
Total	16	8	8	24	18	9	17	7	6
Table n	5815	236	448	3039	184	315	4738	254	471

( ) = based on 25 or fewer unweighted cases.

Table 6.13   Percent with Fair or Poor Health and Mean
Total Non-Hospital Disability Days by
Insurance Coverage and Poverty Level for
the U.S. Population and CHP Subsample
(Under 65).

INSURANCE / POVERTY LEVEL	FAIR OR POOR HEALTH	TOTAL NON-HOSPITAL DISABILITY DAYS
U.S. POPULATION		
Uninsured:		
Equal to or Below 1.5 Poverty	25%	15 days
Above 1.5 Poverty	(15)	9
Insured	14	12
CHP POPULATION		
Uninsured:		
Equal to or Below 1.5 Poverty	20	16
Above 1.5 Poverty	(10)	6
Insured	12	13

( ) = based on 25 or fewer unweighted cases.

Chapter 7
Actual Access to Care

LU ANN ADAY

IN THIS CHAPTER we will examine actual access indicators for selected subgroups in the 1982 national survey. Of particular interest are measures of convenience, utilization, and satisfaction for individuals who have different types of care and coverage and for potentially policy vulnerable race and income groups. These analyses help set the stage for examining who seems to have the least access, based on a "bird's eye" national perspective. The analyses in the chapters that follow provide a closer look at who has what types of care and coverage and why and what their resultant access appears to be.

Convenience

As indicated in Figure 1.1 (Chapter 1), the convenience of care is one indicator of actual access. Table 7.1 provides estimates for selected subgroups on one widely used indicator of convenience — the average time spent waiting before a doctor can actually be seen. Office waiting time has been found to have a significant impact on patients' level of satisfaction with a variety of aspects of their care (Aday, et al., 1980).

The average waiting time overall was around half an hour. Regular hospital outpatient department (OPD) and emergency room (ER) users averaged waits of closer to an hour (49 minutes and 47 minutes), respectively, while those who were more likely to use private doctors waited less than half an hour (25 minutes). This may reflect the fact that OPD and ER users are less apt to have appointments in advance of their visit, which adds substantially to their waiting time (Aday, et al., 1980).

People with public coverage only tended to average longer waits (37 minutes) than those with some form of private insurance (26 to 29 minutes). For those who have the benefit of public insurance, direct costs may be low, but the indirect costs of prolonged waits before being seen may be high.

The findings for different race and income groups bear out that minorities and the poor tend to average the longest waiting times. We saw earlier (Chapter 5) that these groups are more likely than majority White and non-poor individuals to use hospital OPDs and ERs and have some form of public insurance or reduced price source of care.

Utilization

Measures of convenience provide evidence of probable barriers to the receipt of care. The proof of access, however, may be said to be whether or not services are actually received. The tables that follow provide an indication of whether or not certain services are obtained and at what rate.

Table 7.2 summarizes the proportion of the U.S. population and selected subgroups who had at least one visit to a physician in the year. Approximately eight out of ten Americans (81 percent) saw a doctor at least once. Those who had no regular source of care or who routinely used hospital ERs when they needed care had much lower rates of contact — 61 and 69 percent, respectively. Those with some form of insurance coverage seemed to fare well relative to the national average, unlike the uninsured for whom the proportion seeing a physician was lower (70 percent).

These care and coverage factors appear to be more important than race and income *per se* in predicting who sees a doctor. In the past minorities and low-income individuals were much less likely to have been to a doctor than majority Whites and the non-poor.

With the advent of Medicare and Medicaid in the mid-1960s, the use rates of the traditionally disadvantaged groups increased substantially (Aday, et al., 1980). The data in Table 7.2 bear out that there are no significant differences overall in the rates of contacting a doctor by race and income. Poor and minority individuals tend to have poorer health (NCHS, 1985). In the next chapter, we will examine these physician contact rates, controlling for need, to see if these similar use rates are also "equitable" relative to need.

The physician contact rates reported in Table 7.2 refer simply to whether or not a physician was seen at all in a year. These initial contact rates are most apt to be affected by the predisposing, enabling, and need characteristics of the individual patient. Volume measures of use, however, refer to the total number of visits in a given period of time and are influenced both by patient characteristics and predispositions, as well as physician decision-making regarding recommended re-visits and referrals.

There were an average of 6.1 visits for those who had contacted a physician in the year. People who did not have a regular source of medical care tended to average the lowest number of visits (4.7), while those who used OPDs averaged the largest number (7.5). People with public coverage, including the elderly on Medicare, reported over nine visits on average. Visits for those with no insurance or some type of private coverage only more closely approximated the national average. There were no significant differences by race in the number of visits reported. People whose family income was more than 150 percent above the poverty level tended to average fewer visits a year than those with poverty level or near poverty-level incomes.

Table 7.2 also enables a look at the proportion of total ambulatory care visits that are to hospital OPDs or ERs. Around 18 percent of visits overall are to these settings. The proportions are, of course, higher for individuals who regularly use OPDs (49 percent) or ERs (47 percent). Rates of ER and OPD use also tend to be higher for Blacks (27 percent) and the poor (26 percent), who we saw earlier (Chapter 5) are much more likely to use these hospital-based settings regularly.

Hospitalizations represent the most expensive type of health services utilization. It is also generally the least discretionary in that illnesses requiring hospitalization are most often severe ones as well. With the advent of diagnosis related groups (DRGs) under Medicare there is concern being expressed, as indicated in Chapter 1, about the impact of this system of prospective pricing on patterns of hospital admissions and lengths-of-stay.

Table 7.3 provides estimates of the proportion of different groups that were hospitalized in the year and, of those hospitalized, their mean number of days in the hospital, as well as the proportion inpatient use represents of the total services consumed in the year.

About one out of ten people (10 percent) were hospitalized. The rates were much lower for people without a regular source of care (4 percent) or insurance coverage (6 percent). Proportions were on the other hand higher for people with some type of public coverage (17 to 18 percent) — a number of whom were the elderly with Medicare. Correspondingly, the average numbers of days in the hospital tended to be lowest for people without a regular source (4.9) or insurance coverage (7.7). Differences by race and income in terms of both hospitalization rates and days were not statistically significant.

Table 7.3 also provides a summary of the proportion of total inpatient and outpatient service units that represent inpatient utilization. The denominator of the proportion is constructed by assigning a weight of 5.3 to each inpatient day to convert it to equivalent ambulatory visit units and adding these adjusted inpatient day and visit estimates. The numerator is the adjusted inpatient days. (See Appendix A for a more detailed discussion of the construction of this measure.)

The findings suggest that inpatient use as a proportion of total service use tends to be lowest for those with no regular source of care or no insurance. Rates are highest for those regularly using ERs. This suggests that a relatively higher proportion of the care eventually rendered to people who use ERs for their "family doctor" tends to be inpatient- rather than outpatient-oriented. These are the individuals that are apt to contribute most to many hospitals' uncompensated care problems.

Visits to a physician may be for illness-related or preventive reasons. Table 7.4 provides data on an indicator of the use of services for illness-related reasons — the use-disability ratio. It is constructed by dividing the mean number of physician visits for those reporting between 1 and 100 disability days in the year by the

mean number of days reported for the respective groups and multiplying the resultant rate by 100. It may be broadly interpreted as
the proportion of disability days for which visits occurred.

Nationally the ratio of visits to disability days was 52, mean-
ing that there was approximately 1 visit relative to every 2 days of
disability. Those who had no regular source of care tended to have
rates lower than the national average (39) as did those who regularly used ERs for their medical care (42), had both public and
private coverage (44), or were uninsured (44). People who had
some other place they routinely went to for medical care or had
some other form of insurance tended to have higher rates of visits
relative to disability days.

Table 7.5 provides estimates of the proportion of adults having a blood pressure check and women who have had a pap smear
or breast exam in the year. These are important indicators of
whether or not appropriate preventive care procedures have been
obtained.

About three-fourths (78 percent) of U.S. adults eighteen and
over had had their blood pressure checked. These rates were much
lower for individuals without a regular source of medical care (56
percent) or insurance (65 percent). The proportion of Hispanics
having such procedures (74 percent) tended to be lower than the
number of Whites (79 percent), and higher proportions of non-
poor (79 percent) had had a blood pressure reading taken than had
the poor (73 percent).

Approximately 60 percent of the women in the United States
had had a pap smear. The proportion of women having pap
smears tend to be lowest for those who have no particular provider
or place they use (52 percent), are publicly insured (46–50 percent)
or uninsured (50 percent). It seems that minority women, for
whom fertility rates and the risks of cervical cancer are greater
than for majority White women, are more likely to have had this
procedure. There continues to be a gradient by income, however,
with higher income women being more likely to have had this
procedure than low–income women. Two-thirds of the women in
the United States (66 percent) had a breast exam in the course of
the year. Rates once again tended to be lowest for those who used
ERs regularly (25 percent), had no regular provider (48 percent) or
were uninsured (49 percent). Patterns by income are comparable

to those observed for pap smears—lower for poor (56 percent) than for non-poor women (68 percent).

Satisfaction

The preceding analyses have provided an indication of the impact of care and coverage, as well as one's race and income, on the convenience and utilization of services. Satisfaction is another important indicator of access, measured in more subjective patient-oriented terms.

Table 7.6 provides estimates of the proportion of individuals who were not completely satisfied with their most recent visit overall or various other aspects (office waiting time and cost). People who used hospital ERs regularly or had no regular source of care tended to be the most dissatisfied with all of these aspects. Rates of dissatisfaction as a whole were highest with the cost of the visit. Around 40 percent of the U.S. population were less than completely satisfied with this aspect of their care.

Table 7.7 provides a somewhat more direct indicator of who had to pay nothing out-of-pocket for their hospital stays—the most costly form of medical care. It shows that about four out of ten people who were hospitalized (43 percent) did not have to pay anything out of their own pocket for their stay. Those who were least likely to pay anything themselves were people who used ERs as their "regular" source of care, only had some form of public coverage and were minority and poor. To the extent that out-of-pocket costs serve as a barrier to obtaining needed hospital services, then the financial access barriers would appear to be less for these individuals. These are, on the other hand, apt to be the groups of most concern to hospital administrators as contributing to the uncompensated or undercompensated care problem in their hospitals, and to the extent they cannot afford to pay, perhaps prime candidates for "dumping" in many institutions.

Summary

This chapter has summarized the actual convenience and utilization of and satisfaction with medical care for the U.S. population. There is evidence that many of the traditional access barriers by race and income *per se* have disappeared. Where one regularly goes for care and the presence of and/or type of third-party coverage continue to be of considerable import in predicting who uses what types of services, to what extent, whether they are convenient or not and how satisfactory the process of care-seeking is found to be.

Table 7.1.   Mean Office Waiting Time for Recent Visit,
for the U.S. Population by Selected
Characteristics.

CHARACTERISTICS	MEAN OFFICE WAITING TIME
Regular Source of Care	
Private Office/Clinic	25 minutes
Hospital OPD	49
Hospital ER	47
Other	28
No Regular Source	30
Insurance Coverage	
Public Only	37
Private Only	26
Public and Private	29
No Insurance	31
Race	
White	25
Black	37
Hispanic	41
Poverty Level	
Less Than Poverty	34
1.0-1.5 Poverty	35
Greater Than 1.5	26
Total	27
Table n	6610

Table 7.2. Percent Seeing a Physician, Mean Visits for
Those with One or More, and Rate of ER
and OPD Use to Total Use the Last Year, for
the U.S. Population by Selected
Characteristics.

CHARACTERISTICS	PERCENT SEEING A PHYSICIAN	MEAN VISITS (1+)	RATE OF ER & OPD TO TOTAL USE
Regular Source of Care			
Private Office/Clinic	84%	6.1	.13
Hospital OPD	86	7.5	.49
Hospital ER	69	6.4	.47
Other	84	6.4	.13
No Regular Source	61	4.7	.24
Insurance Coverage			
Public Only	85	9.6	.23
Private Only	82	5.6	.16
Public and Private	88	7.3	.28
No Insurance	70	6.3	.24
Race			
White	82	5.9	.17
Black	82	6.7	.27
Hispanic	80	6.7	.17
Poverty Level			
Less Than Poverty	78	7.3	.26
1.0-1.5 Poverty	80	7.7	.21
Greater Than 1.5	82	5.7	.15
Total	81	6.1	.18
Table n	6610	5383	5383

Table 7.3.   Percent Hospitalized, Mean Hospital Days
for Those with One or More, and Rate of
Inpatient to Total Use the Last Year, for the
U.S. Population by Selected Characteristics.

CHARACTERISTICS	PERCENT HOSPITALIZED	MEAN HOSPITAL DAYS (1+)	RATE OF INPATIENT TO TOTAL USE
Regular Source of Care			
Private Office/Clinic	10%	9.4 days	.51
Hospital OPD	12	11.5	.54
Hospital ER	15	(29.0)	.83
Other	11	9.4	.49
No Regular Source	4	4.9	.28
Insurance Coverage			
Public Only	17	11.3	.56
Private Only	9	8.9	.47
Public and Private	18	12.7	.66
No Insurance	6	7.7	.35
Race			
White	10	9.8	.52
Black	9	12.3	.51
Hispanic	9	6.5	.36
Poverty Level			
Less Than Poverty	11	10.1	.51
1.0-1.5 Poverty	13	11.7	.57
Greater Than 1.5	9	9.4	.50
Total	10	9.9	.51
Table n	6554	762	5383

─────────

( ) = based on 25 or fewer unweighted cases.

Table 7.4. Use-Disability Ratio, for the U.S. Population by Selected Characteristics.

CHARACTERISTICS	USE-DISABILITY RATIO
Regular Source of Care	
Private Office/Clinic	53
Hospital OPD	54
Hospital ER	42
Other	63
No Regular Source	39
Insurance Coverage	
Public Only	58
Private Only	54
Public and Private	44
No Insurance	44
Race	
White	51
Black	57
Hispanic	58
Poverty Level	
Less Than Poverty	55
1.0-1.5 Poverty	48
Greater Than 1.5	53
Total	52
Table n	3735

Table 7.5.   Percent Adults 18 and Over Having a Blood
             Pressure Check, Women Having a Pap
             Smear, Breast Exam, Within the Last Year,
             for the U.S. Population by Selected
             Characteristics.

CHARACTERISTICS	PERCENT ADULTS 18+ HAVING BLOOD PRESSURE CHECK	PERCENT WOMEN 18+ HAVING PAP SMEAR	PERCENT WOMEN 18+ HAVING BREAST EXAM
Regular Source of Care			
Private Office/Clinic	82%	61%	68%
Hospital OPD	81	71	72
Hospital ER	63	60	25
Other	75	62	68
No Regular Source	56	52	48
Insurance Coverage			
Public Only	83	46	52
Private Only	78	65	70
Public and Private	85	50	65
No Insurance	65	50	49
Race			
White	79	59	66
Black	77	64	67
Hispanic	74	69	64
Poverty Level			
Less Than Poverty	73	53	56
1.0-1.5 Poverty	78	56	63
Greater Than 1.5	79	63	68
Total	78	60	66
Table n	4463	2644	2652

Table 7.6.   Percent Not Completely Satisfied With
Aspects of Recent Visit, for the U.S.
Population by Selected Characteristics.

CHARACTERISTICS	PERCENT NOT COMPLETELY SATISFIED WITH ...		
	VISIT OVERALL	OFFICE WAITING TIME	OUT-OF- POCKET COSTS
Regular Source of Care			
Private Office/Clinic	20%	29%	41%
Hospital OPD	29	40	34
Hospital ER	43	45	45
Other	21	29	26
No Regular Source	37	42	47
Insurance Coverage			
Public Only	21	26	26
Private Only	23	33	42
Public and Private	15	23	35
No Insurance	32	37	46
Race			
White	21	31	40
Black	28	34	43
Hispanic	28	37	39
Poverty Level			
Less Than Poverty	26	31	38
1.0-1.5 Poverty	25	37	43
Greater Than 1.5	21	31	41
Total	23	31	40
Table n	4671	4680	4537

Table 7.7.   Percent With No Out-of-Pocket Costs for Hospital Stay, for the U.S. Population by Selected Characteristics.

CHARACTERISTICS	PERCENT WITH NO OUT-OF-POCKET COSTS FOR HOSPITAL STAY
Regular Source of Care	
Private Office/Clinic	41%
Hospital OPD	60
Hospital ER	(93)
Other	50
No Regular Source	(15)
Insurance Coverage	
Public Only	82
Private Only	35
Public and Private	57
No Insurance	24
Race	
White	42
Black	46
Hispanic	48
Poverty Level	
Less Than Poverty	50
1.0-1.5 Poverty	46
Greater Than 1.5	41
Total	43
Table n	556

( ) = based on 25 or fewer unweighted cases.

Chapter 8
Multivariate Analysis of Access to Care

MEEI-SHIA CHEN
CHRISTOPHER S. LYTTLE

IN PREVIOUS CHAPTERS, we examined need for and access to medical care by persons with different regular sources of care and insurance coverage. This was done mainly using bivariate analyses.

In this chapter, based on multivariate analyses of the national sample, we will examine the impact of many of these variables simultaneously. We will explore the relative importance of various determinants of individuals' selection of different sources of care or insurance and their ultimate access to care. The major questions to be addressed in this chapter are: (1) Who has what type of care and insurance coverage; (2) Are the differences in access to medical care for groups who choose different regular sources of care and insurance coverage due primarily to equitable or inequitable factors; and (3) What is the relative importance of various equitable and inequitable variables in accounting for differences in access among these groups?

Equitable factors refer to measures of need as well as predisposing variables which are highly correlated with need (e.g., age, sex). Immutable inequitable factors refer to other predisposing (e.g., education of family head, time in community) or enabling system (e.g., residence, per capita income) variables* that are not

---

*MDs per one thousand is included as an immutable inequitable variable, because (1) from the consumers' point of view, relative to regular source of care and insurance coverage it is a less immediate indicator of potential access to care, and (2) there are indications in the literature that it may or may not be directly associated with consumers' *ultimate* access to care in a community (Andersen and Aday, 1978).

readily altered by health policy, while mutable inequitable factors focus on the more immediate "means" for obtaining services, based on one's regular source of care or insurance coverage (Figure 1.1).

Who Has What Type of Care and Coverage?

Before inspecting the access to medical care of different regular source and insurance groups we want to look systematically at who has which types of care and coverage. In Tables 8.1 and 8.2 we describe and compare the groups with or without various regular sources of care and insurance coverage on a range of equitable and inequitable variables. This is done using multiple regression analyses of dummy coded (having a type of care or insurance vs. not having it, 1 vs. 0) dependent variables. Each dependent variable is regressed on the various equitable and inequitable variables. Some categorical independent variables are also dummy coded. For example, for sex male is coded as 1 and female is coded as 0; for ethnicity Whites is the reference group compared with Blacks, Hispanics, and other races. Region, residence, insurance coverage, and regular source of care are treated as dummy variables with "East," "suburban," "private insurance only," and "private doctor" as the reference groups. Perceived health, occupation of household head, and poverty level are coded so that more positive values represent *better* perceived health, *higher* status (i.e. white collar) occupations and *higher* income levels, respectively. The remaining variables are simple volume measures. Analyses of insurance coverage are made separately for those under sixty-five and those sixty-five and over since practically all people sixty-five and over are covered by Medicare. Betas and their significance levels* indicate the relative importance of the respective independent variables in explaining whether or not one has a certain regular source of care or insurance. It should be stressed here that all independent variables are analyzed simultaneously. Therefore, the

---

*It should be noted that all t's in all the analyses of this chapter are adjusted down by dividing them by the highest design effect of the variables involved in the analysis. (See Appendix B.) Further, the unweighted rather than weighted n is used for the relevant degrees of freedom. These adjustments are incorporated to reflect the fact that the sample was weighted and non-random (clustered).

beta of each variable represents its effect on the dependent variable with the other variables held constant.

Regular Source of Care

We saw in Chapter 5 that a majority of Americans (74 percent) named a private office or clinic as their regular source of care. What kind of people are they? Are they different from those who do not regularly use private doctors?

The betas for equitable and inequitable variables in the first column of Table 8.1 indicate the characteristics of people who use private doctors as their regular source of care. The regular users of private office or clinics are much more likely to be females than males (beta = -.087, p < .001). We saw in Chapter 6 that regular users of private physicians and those who could identify no regular source of care have better health than the users of other types of care. Indeed, we found perceived health a positive predictor (beta = .036, p < .01) of having or not having private doctors when other variables are not controlled (data not shown in table). But after controlling for other variables, especially occupational and poverty levels, perceived health becomes an insignificant predictor. In other words, higher occupational and income levels rather than better perceived health seem to be the underlying reasons for an individual to use private doctors for their regular care. Having better health status does not seem to predict that people will choose private doctors for their regular care, after other equitable and inequitable variables are taken into account.

Whites, in comparison with Blacks and other races, are more likely to name private doctors as their regular source of care. People with private physicians are also more likely to be employed and have higher occupational (beta = .087, p < .001) and income levels (beta = .039, p < .01). Unemployment status is coded as "no occupation." Interestingly, education is not a significant predictor. One may infer that occupation, employment, and income are predictive of individuals' using private doctors probably because of the fact that being employed or having a higher income better enables them to pay for the services of a private medical provider. Additionally, the longer an individual has been in the community, the more likely that they will have a private doctor as a regular source of care (beta = .123, p < .001).

The negative, and significant beta (beta = -.056, p < .001) for the number of physicians per one thousand population reflects the fact that people who use private doctors tend to reside in areas that have lower physician to population ratios. We also find that residents of central cities are less likely than those from suburban areas (beta = -.061, p < .001) to use private doctors. Central cities may have relatively large numbers of physicians who are highly specialized and work in medical schools and large teaching hospitals. Residents of these areas may, however, have access to fewer private practice physicians (Andersen & Aday, 1978). Residents of non-SMSA areas are also less likely than those of suburban areas to regularly use private office/clinics (beta = -.037, p < .01). This, on the other hand, suggests the fewer number of private doctors in these areas. As for region, people in the West are significantly less likely to use private doctors for their regular care.

The kind of insurance coverage one has may play an important role in determining whether the person has a regular source of care and what that source might be. Having some type of private insurance is associated with using private doctors regularly for care. Those having only public insurance (beta = -.029, p < .05) or no insurance coverage (beta = -.120, p < .001) are much less likely to use private doctors.

Examining the betas for the predictors of who regularly use hospital outpatient departments (OPDs), we find regular hospital OPD users are quite different from those who regularly go to private doctors. OPD users tend to perceive their health status to be poorer. Blacks (beta = .059, p < .001) were more likely than Whites to be regular hospital OPD users. They also tend to have lower occupational levels (beta = -.074, p < .001). In contrast to those who see private doctors, hospital OPD users tend to be newer to the community (beta = -.053, p < .001) and residents of central city areas (beta = .061, p < .001) or farm areas (beta = .050, p < .001). Hospital OPDs are less popular in the South as a regular source of care than in the East (beta = -.033, p < .05). The individuals who do not have some private insurance, i.e., those who have only public insurance or have no insurance coverage, are more likely to report hospital OPDs as their regular source of care.

Turning to the third column of Table 8.1, the significant predictors demonstrate that regular hospital emergency room (ER) users tend to be male (beta = .046, p < .001) and Black (beta

= .036, p < .01), and report more non-bed disability days on average (beta = .038, p < .001). The model explained a very small portion of the variance (0.9 percent), however.

The utilization of hospital ERs has grown tremendously in the last thirty years or more. Studies have suggested that much of the usage of hospital ERs are for the treatment of nonurgent problems (Straus, et al., 1983; Stratmann and Ullman, 1975, Ullman, et al., 1975; Davidson, 1978). Davidson (1978) indicated that there are many reasons for the usage of ERs. Many studies have found that the lack of accessibility to other sources is one major reason (White and O'Connor, 1970; Roth, 1971; Jacobs and Thurber, 1972). Davidson (1978) concluded from the review of studies on ER users that some are more likely to use ERs because they do not have family doctors for care and others use them when their family doctors are not available. Ullman et al. (1975) found in their study of the ER patients at an urban community hospital that the majority of ER patients used ERs very infrequently and the multiple users were more likely to be Blacks, low-income, and from inner city areas.

In the 1977 National Medical Care Expenditure Survey (NMCES), 1 percent of the sample reported an ER as their usual source of care (Kasper and Barrish, 1982). The results of this survey did not show significant variation among those who reported an ER as their regular source in terms of their age, sex, family income, education level, perceived health status, residence, or region. The NMCES data did confirm that there were somewhat higher proportions of Blacks, Hispanics, and Medicaid recipients among regular ER users, however.

Five percent of the national sample used other clinics, including mostly government clinics and some company/union and school clinics. Multivariate analysis of this group vs. other groups demonstrates that they tend to be younger (beta = -.029, p < .05), Blacks (beta = .049, p < .001), and have lower occupational levels (beta = -.073, p < .001) and incomes (beta = -.033, p < .05). They also tend to be new to the community and live in areas where the number of physicians per one thousand population is higher (beta = .090, p < .001) and the per capita family income is lower (beta = -.039, p < .05). People from the North Central (beta = .038, p < .05) and West (beta = .035, p < .05) regions, compared with those in the East, tend to use these clinics.

The results of comparing those without a regular source of care with those having some type of regular source of care are shown in the last column of Table 8.1. Those who do not have a regular source of care tend to be older (beta = .060, p < .001). This may reflect the fact that children are more likely than adults to have a regular source of care. They also tend to be male (beta = .080, p < . 001). They perceive their health to be better (beta = .055, p < .001) and have fewer bed days (beta = -.027, p < .05). In addition, they tend to be poorly-educated (beta = -.043, p < .01) and newcomers to the community (beta = -.087, p < .001). As has been found in previous studies (Aday, et al., 1980; Aday, et al., 1984), one of the major reasons for not having a regular source of care is that the family has just moved and may not have had a chance to locate a regular source of care. Another strong predictor is the fact that they do not have insurance coverage (beta = .103, p < .001). However, having both public and private insurance (beta = -.038, p < .01) as opposed to having private insurance only decreases the possibility of having no regular source of care.

It should be noted that the above-described models for analyzing having or not having various regular sources of care account for a small percent (less than 7.8) of the variance for each dependent variable. Therefore, to better understand the reasons for an individual's having or not having various regular sources of care, we need to study other variables than those included in our analysis, such as respondents' attitudes and beliefs toward medical care in general or physicians in particular.

Insurance Coverage

Table 8.2 shows the betas and the significance levels for equitable and inequitable variables predicting whether or not an individual would have various types of insurance coverage. The first four columns of Table 8.2 indicate the results of the analyses for those under sixty-five, and the last column for those sixty-five and over.

Public insurance for those under sixty-five principally includes people on Medicaid. Although a relatively large proportion of those with public insurance are children, age was not a significant factor in predicting having public insurance, controlling for other factors. People with public insurance only also have poor perceived health (beta = -.033, p < .05) and a greater number of disability days (beta for non-bed disability days = .039, p < .01; beta for bed days = .093, p < .001).

Surprisingly, there was no significant ethnic difference for having or not having public insurance only. In Chapter 5, we found that persons with public insurance include a larger proportion of Blacks and Hispanics. Upon further examination by hierarchical multiple regression analyses (data not shown in table), we find, indeed, Blacks (beta = .089, p < .001) and Hispanics (beta = .024, p < .05), in contrast with whites, are significantly more likely to have public insurance only, *if their educational, occupational, and poverty levels are not controlled.* However, after controlling for these variables, the magnitudes of betas for Blacks or Hispanics vs. whites becomes insignificant. This suggests that "being minority" is only the apparent factor for Blacks and Hispanics to have public insurance. On the other hand, the significant underlying reasons are their lower occupational levels and the fact that they are more likely to be unemployed (beta = -.076, p < .001) and poor (beta = -.181, p < .001). In fact, poverty level is the strongest predictor among all the variables included in the analysis for having or not having public insurance coverage.

Those who have public insurance only are relatively new to the community (beta = -.026, p < .05). They also tend to be from communities with greater numbers of physicians per one thousand population. Again, this may be the effect of large medical centers or teaching hospitals where there are larger concentrations of physicians. In terms of region, southern residents are underrepresented in this group (beta = -.056, p < .001). People with public insurance only are also more likely to use hospital OPDs (beta = .039, p < .01).

As mentioned earlier, a majority (83 percent) of the U.S. population under sixty-five have private insurance only. It would be interesting to compare this group of people with those from the other 17 percent of the population. Table 8.2 (second column) shows the results of the comparison. There is no age or sex difference between these two groups. The significant betas for need variables clearly demonstrate that people with private insurance only have much better health status. They perceive their health as being better and have fewer disability days.

Hispanics (beta = -.026, p < .05) and other races (beta = -.024, p < .05) are less likely to have private insurance than

Whites. However, Blacks are not significantly different from Whites in this respect. Without controlling for education, occupation, and poverty level simultaneously (data not shown in the table), the minority population including Blacks (beta = -.071, p < .001), Hispanics (beta = -.060, p < .001) and other races (beta = -.043, p < .001) are significantly less likely to use private insurance only. However, controlling for education, occupation, and poverty level, we find the changes in the magnitude of the effect: the beta for Blacks vs. Whites becomes insignificant and those for Hispanics and other races decrease. As in the case of the public only insurance group, "blackness" is only the apparent reason for their not being able to purchase private insurance. The major contributing factors are their lower educational (beta = .038, p < .01), occupational (beta = .088, p < .001) and poverty (beta = .316, p < .001) levels. People from central cities (beta = -.051, p < .001), non-SMSA areas (beta = -.032, p < .05) or the western region of the country (beta = -.034, p < .05) are less likely to have private insurance only.

Those who use private doctors regularly are more likely, than those who use other sources of care and those who do not have regular source of care, to have private insurance only. However, having private insurance may be the determinant of an individual's use of private doctors, rather than vice versa.

There are fewer significant predictors for persons having or not having both public and private insurance, as shown in the third column of Table 8.2. These predictors indicate that, when examining all variables simultaneously, being older (beta = .028, p < .05), having more non-bed disability days (beta = .083, p < .001), being Black (beta = .051, p < .001), having a lower occupational status (beta = -.061, p < .001), and being poor (beta = -.077, p < .001) are important in predicting whether or not an individual has both public and private insurance. In addition, people from the western region of the country are less likely than those from the East to have both public and private insurance. Residents of non-SMSA areas, as opposed to suburban areas, tend to have both public and private insurance (beta = .033, p < .05).

As mentioned in Chapter 5, eleven percent of the people under sixty-five are uninsured. Who are they? What could lead them to be uninsured? The fourth column of Table 8.2 attempts to answer these questions. The findings on need variables are mixed:

while the uninsured have poorer perceived health, they have fewer non-bed disability days than the insured. The significant and negative beta for the dummy variable "Black vs. White" (beta $= -.059$, $p < .001$) reveals that, all other variables being equal, Blacks would be less likely to be uninsured than Whites. Hispanics would have a somewhat greater possibility of being uninsured than Whites (beta $= .027$, $p < .05$). As in previous analyses, we examined the effect of ethnicity and found that, without controlling for other variables (data not shown in tables), Hispanics (beta $= .070$, $p < .001$) and Blacks (beta $= .027$, $p < .05$) are more likely than Whites to be uninsured. The apparent phenomenon for Blacks changes after the adjustment for other variables, especially poverty level (beta $= -.247$, $p < .001$). The effect of being Hispanic also decreases. Poverty level is an extremely important factor that accounts for an individual being uninsured.

Those without insurance tend to be from lower income communities (beta $= -.034$, $p < .05$) or central cities (beta $= .035$, $p < .01$). People from the western and southern regions are more likely to be uninsured. In comparison with those who routinely use private doctors, regular hospital OPD users (beta $= .070$, $p < .001$) or hospital ER users (beta $= .028$, $p < .05$) are more likely to have no insurance. As one would have expected, those who have no regular source of care also tend to be uninsured (beta for "None vs. Private M.D." $= .111$, $p < .001$).

The last column of Table 8.2 shows the results comparing the characteristics of people sixty-five and over who have public insurance only with those who have public insurance and supplementary private insurance. Interestingly, there are few significant predictors, suggesting that these two groups are quite similar in many aspects, such as age, sex, length of time in the community, residence, region, and disability days. The significant predictors indicate that the elderly with public insurance only are more likely, than those who also have supplementary private insurance, to be Hispanics (beta $= .141$, $p < .001$), have lower income levels (beta $= -.178$, $p < .001$), have no regular source of care (beta $= .099$, $p < .01$) and have poorer perceived health (beta $= -.084$, $p < .05$).

In comparison with the analysis for regular source of care, the models used for predicting whether or not an individual would have various types of insurance coverage account for a much larger proportion of variance. With the exception of the analysis for public and private insurance which only contributes to 3.9 percent of the variance, the equitable and inequitable variables account for more than nine percent of the variance, suggesting that these variables are fairly important in predicting an individual's having various types of insurance coverage.

Are Access Differences by Care and Coverage Equitable or Inequitable?

The previous analyses have provided us with a description and comparison of groups with different types of regular source of care and insurance coverage. In this section, we examine the differences in medical access between these groups to determine whether these observed differences are primarily a function of their respective need for care (reflecting an equitable system) or due to inequitable factors — which may or may not be mutable to (manipulable by) health policy. Multiple regression analyses with hierarchical modelling are used to address this question.

Need variables including perceived health, non-bed disability days, and bed days as well as age and sex (which can be used as proxies of need because of their high correlation with health) are entered first. If the differences in access measures are primarily attributable to need, age, and sex, then a more equitable system may be said to exist. Inequitable variables that are immutable to health policy, such as ethnicity, education, poverty level, employment, are entered next. Either regular source of care or insurance coverage, an inequitable but mutable variable, is entered in the last step. This will enable a look at whether the differences between subgroups can be explained by differences in their various sources of care or insurance coverage — factors which may be altered by changes in the organization and financing of care.

The access outcome variables examined in this section include physician utilization (whether or not a doctor was seen and the average number of visits), hospital utilization (admission to the hospital and hospital days in a year), preventive services (having a blood pressure checkup, pap smear, or breast exam), and satisfaction with their recent visit to a physician overall (percent not completely satisfied). Unadjusted and adjusted means or percentages, betas, and significance levels are obtained in each step. Note that "private doctor," "private only" (for under sixty-five), and "public and private" (for sixty-five and over) groups do not have betas because they are treated as reference groups in the analysis. These statistics (shown in Tables 8.3 to 8.10) enable us to compare subgroups of interest on these access measures after adjusting for equitable or inequitable variables in each step. Independent variables to be entered in the hierarchical model are somewhat different for different access variables. The criteria for selecting variables to control are (1) their theoretical relevance based on existing literature or their correspondence with existing health policy concerns, and (2) their empirical (i.e., significant) correlation with the access measures studied. The independent variables included in the analysis according to the first criterion (regardless of the significance of their correlation) are need, age, sex, ethnicity, poverty level, insurance coverage, and regular source of care. The additional variables included due to their significant correlation with each access variable are education of head for physician contact and visits, education of respondent for the three preventive services, employment status of head, time in community, and residence for physician contact, and per capita income for physician visits.

Physician Utilization

Table 8.3 shows the results of the analysis on percent seeing a physician in the last year. The unadjusted percentage by regular source of care indicates that the regular hospital ER users (beta = -.050, p < .001) and those without a regular source of care (beta = -.187, p < .001) were significantly less likely to have seen a physician in the last year. While 84 to 86 percent of the regular users of private doctors, hospital OPDs, or other clinics reported going to a physician last year, only 69 percent of hospital ER users and even a smaller 61 percent of the "no regular source" group did so. The small changes in the adjusted percentages and betas in the adjustment process further demonstrate that very little of the difference is attributable to equitable or other inequitable variables. Even after all the adjustments, significant differences continue to persist. This finding suggests that the lack of a regular source of care or going to ERs regularly for care tends to inhibit the individual (regardless of needs, socioeconomic status, or insurance coverage) from seeking a physician's care.

Among various insurance groups for people under sixty-five years of age, those with public insurance only are more likely to have seen a physician (90 percent, beta = .032, p < .01). However, this is principally due to equitable characteristics since the difference becomes insignificant after adjusting for these variables. This result suggests that Medicaid or Medicare help make the entry to physician services easier for the recipients who *need* them.

On the other hand, the uninsured are much less likely to have seen a physician (70 percent, beta = −.091, p < .001). Need, age, or sex explain a very minor portion of this difference. Inequitable variables contribute to part of the inequity; there is a 2 percent increase after adjusting for immutable inequitable variables (mostly due to their lower income level) and another 2 percent increase after adjusting for regular source of care. The inequity for the uninsured continues to exist after all these adjustments, however.

The unadjusted percentage seeing a physician for people sixty-five and over is 89 percent for those with both public and private insurance and 81 percent for those with public insurance only. The elderly without supplementary private insurance are significantly less likely to have seen a physician during the year. The adjustment process reveals that their lack of a regular source of care contributes to part (2 percent) of the difference.

Shown in Table 8.4 are the results of the analysis on mean visits for those who have seen a physician within the last year. The unadjusted number of visits are 6.07 for private doctor users, 7.48 for hospital OPD users, 6.43 for hospital ER users, 6.44 for other clinic users, and 4.74 for those without a regular source of care. Hospital OPD users have significantly more visits (beta = .037, p < .01). However, this is only apparent because it becomes insignificant after the adjustment for need — regular hospital OPD users make more physician visits due to their greater need. Those who do not have a regular source of care have significantly fewer visits (beta = −.036, p < .01), mostly due to their lower level of needs, as their mean number of visits increases (5.27) and the beta becomes insignificant after adjusting for need, suggesting if their need were more like the rest of the population (higher) their average number of visits would be higher, too.

The mean number of visits is significantly higher for those under sixty-five with some public insurance (12.74 for the public insurance only group and 8.88 for the public and private insurance group as opposed to 5.63 for the private insurance only group and

6.32 for the uninsured). The greater number of visits of those with both public and private insurance is a function of their higher level of needs, as the number of visits decreases and the beta become insignificant, after controlling for equitable variables. Although a major part of the variation for those who have public insurance only is due to their greater needs, the difference continues to exist after adjustments. As mentioned in previous studies (Aday et al., 1984), this overutilization may reflect the tendency of physicians to encourage those with public insurance only to return for follow-up care more often than people with private insurance or those with no insurance coverage at all. Or, on the contrary, it may reflect doctor shopping or discontinuous or poorly coordinated follow-up care (for those in the Medicaid and Medicare programs).

The average number of visits is 6.68 for people over sixty-five with both public and private insurance and 6.49 for those with public insurance only (Table 8.4). This difference is not significant. Adjusting for need, we still find insignificant differences between them.

Hospital Utilization

Table 8.5 shows the percent hospitalized in the last year adjusted for equitable and inequitable variables for subgroups with or without a regular source of care and insurance coverage. Only 4 percent of those without a regular source of care were hospitalized, which was significantly lower (beta = -.063, p < .001) than those who had a regular provider. Part of this lower admission rate is a function of their lower need, since adjustment for the equitable variables results in a 2 percent increase. The difference continues to exist after all adjustments have been made. As in the case of physician contact, having no regular source of care is an important barrier to an individual's admission to the hospital. Therefore, to improve the equity of hospitalization, linking of individuals to a regular medical care provider would seem to facilitate access to this important source of care.

Very high proportions of people under sixty-five with some public insurance were hospitalized last year (20 percent for the public insurance only group and 17 percent for the public and private insurance group), compared to those with the private insurance only (9 percent) and the uninsured (6 percent). However, their greater needs are responsible for a large part of the excessive use: adjustments for need, age, and sex reduce the difference by 4 to 8 percent (a reduction to 12 to 13 percent being hospitalized). Even after all adjustments there is still a significantly higher proportion hospitalized in the public and private insurance group, as shown in its significant beta (.026, $p < .05$) and larger percent (13) being hospitalized, compared with the private insurance only group (9 percent). This may suggest that having both public and private insurance encourages more admissions to the hospital. As expected, the uninsured have a significantly lower hospitalization rate — only 6 percent (beta $= -.030$, $p < .05$). This association becomes even stronger after adjustment, suggesting the importance of not having insurance as a deterrent to hospitalization.

For people sixty-five and over, those with both public and private insurance have a higher (but insignificant) proportion (19 percent) hospitalized within the last year compared to those with public insurance only (15 percent). This difference changes little after adjustment.

Mean hospital days for those hospitalized within the last year, by regular source of care and insurance coverage, are shown in Table 8.6. Mean hospital days, the betas and significance levels were obtained based on log-transformed hospital days to avoid biased results resulting from a skewed distribution of hospital days. However, the unadjusted unlogged hospital days are also shown in the table. Hospital ER users have an average of 28.97 hospital days as opposed to 9.41 days for those who use private doctors. However, there were fewer than twenty-five regular hospital ER users in this sample.

Those without a regular source of care have significantly fewer hospital days (4.86). This difference is partially attributable to their lower level of needs, as revealed by the decrease of significance level after controlling for equitable variables. Even with all the variables controlled, having no regular source of care results in a significantly shorter stay in the hospital in comparison with having some regular source of care.

For those under sixty-five, people who have both public and private insurance have a greater number of hospital days (20.56) than any of the other insurance coverage categories. Part of their excessive number of hospital days is due to their greater need; with adjustments for need, age, and sex the gap of logged hospital days between these people and those with private insurance only is narrowed, and the magnitude of the beta (.095, p < .01) is smaller. However, the difference exists even after adjustments for equitable and inequitable variables. Therefore, having both public and private insurance encourages not only hospital admissions but also increases the number of days hospitalized once admitted. The lack of insurance tends to shorten the individual's stay in the hospital; those who have no insurance have only 7.74 mean hospital days. This difference becomes even more pronounced after controlling for need (beta = -.125, p < .001), as well as the other inequitable adjustments.

For those sixty-five and over, people with only public insurance have more mean hospital days (12.27) than those with public and private insurance (9.99). This difference is more pronounced after controlling for equitable variables (beta = .206, p < .01) and persists after all adjustments. This result differs from that of the analysis for those under sixty-five; those under sixty-five with private and public insurance have more hospital days. The latter, as mentioned earlier, are often people who become eligible for Medicaid by "spending down" their personal resources until they qualify. This is then reflected in their longer hospital stays.

Preventive Services

Table 8.7 shows the percent of adults having a blood pressure check within the last year according to regular source of care and insurance coverage. Users of hospital OPDs and those using a private doctor are similar in their rates of receiving blood pressure checks (81 and 82 percent). However, regular users of hospital ERs, users of other clinics, and those with no regular source of care are all less likely to have had a blood pressure check (64 percent, beta = -.058, p < .001; 75 percent, beta = -.039, p < .01 and 56 percent, beta = -.212, p < .001). These inequities still exist after adjustments. This is not surprising because the possibility of having one's blood pressure checked is much lower if one has not developed a relationship with a specific health care provider.

The analysis by insurance coverage for people under sixty-five indicates that among the uninsured a significantly lower proportion have had a blood pressure check than is the case for the insured (65 as opposed to 78 to 81 percent). Immutable variables including ethnicity, education, employment, and poverty level are responsible for part of the inequity. A lack of a regular source of care also contributes to the inequity. Therefore, having both a regular source of care and insurance coverage are important factors affecting whether an adult is likely to have had a blood pressure check in the last year. Finally, a lower proportion of those sixty-five and over with public insurance only (84 percent) have had a blood pressure check, compared with those with both public and private insurance. Although, the difference is not significant, the adjustment shows that the difference is primarily due to the former's lack of a regular source of care, as the difference is eliminated after controlling for this variable.

The percentages of adult women who have had a pap smear within the last year, according to regular source of care and insurance coverage, are shown in Table 8.8. A greater proportion (71 percent) of regular hospital OPD users have had a pap smear. This proportion becomes even larger (73 percent) after controlling for needs. This reflects that hospital OPDs appear more likely to provide their clients pap smear services. As expected, a smaller proportion (52 percent, beta = -.052, p < .01) of those without a regular source of care than those private doctor users (60 percent) receive a pap smear. Adjustments for equitable variables reveal an even lower proportion (48 percent) of this group having pap smears, which is partially due to their socioeconomic status and lack of insurance.

Similar to the pattern for blood pressure checks, a smaller proportion of uninsured women under sixty-five had a pap smear (50 percent), and this underutilization exists even after adjusting for equitable and inequitable variables. A higher proportion of women sixty-five and over with both public and private insurance (45 percent) have had a pap smear compared to those with public insurance only (37 percent). Although the difference is not significant, it continues to exist after adjustment.

Table 8.9 shows the percentage of adult women having a breast exam within the last year, adjusted for equitable and inequitable variables, according to regular source of care and insurance coverage. The pattern is very similar to that of blood pressure checks: even with needs and inequitable variables controlled, women who regularly use hospital ERs are less likely to have had a breast exam. Hospital ERs are, of course, less likely to provide routine preventive services than are other health care facilities. In addition, women with no regular source of care or insurance are less likely to have had a breast exam, compared to those with a regular source or coverage. Furthermore, for those sixty-five and over, a significantly lower proportion of women with public insurance only have had a breast exam. The 3 percent increase after adjusting for regular source of care indicates that the difference is partially attributable to their lack of a regular source of care.

Overall Satisfaction with Most Recent Visit

In the preceding analyses, we have examined access to medical care among groups according to their regular source of care and insurance coverage. Satisfaction is another dimension of access from the consumer's perspective. As shown in Table 8.10, in comparison with those who routinely use private doctors, regular hospital OPD and ER users are much less likely to be satisfied. Thirty percent of the former and 43 percent of the latter are less than completely satisfied with their most recent visit overall, as opposed to 20 percent for the private doctor users. The variation in these two groups is in part attributable to their greater health needs (2 percent decrease after adjustment). The difference remains significant even after controlling for equitable and inequitable variables. This may suggest that hospital facilities provide less satisfactory services to their clients than private office/clinics. A large proportion of those without a regular source of care (37 percent) are also not completely satisfied with their last visit overall. This is not due to their need, age, or sex, as the percentage remains the same after adjusting for those variables. Inequitable variables examined here explain only a small part of the difference.

The analysis of satisfaction in terms of insurance coverage shows that the uninsured under sixty-five are significantly more likely to be less than completely satisfied (32 percent, beta = .060, $p < .001$). This is in large part attributable to their lack of a regular source of care since the difference becomes smaller ($p < .05$) after adjusting for this variable. Nevertheless, the uninsured tend to be less than satisfied with their visits overall regardless of their equitable or inequitable characteristics. The two insurance groups over sixty-five are not much different in their satisfaction levels as indicated by similar percentages being not completely satisfied.

Which Factors Are Most Important in Predicting Access?

In the previous section, we discussed whether the observed differences in medical access between the groups with or without regular source or insurance coverage are attributable to equitable or inequitable variables. In this section, we examine further the relative importance of these variables, as well as regular source of care and insurance coverage, in explaining individual's utilization of and satisfaction with health services. This can be addressed by comparing the betas and the significance levels of t's that result from the multiple regression of equitable and inequitable variables on each access measure (see Tables 8.11 for those under sixty-five and Table 8.12 for those sixty-five and over).

Physician Utilization

Physician contact is an important access measure. It can be studied to assess who gets into the medical system and who does not. Table 8.11 shows that for people under sixty-five, there are several significant predictors. Most equitable variables and some inequitable variables including education of head, living on a farm, having no regular source of care or insurance coverage, are strong predictors ($p < .001$). The negative beta ($-.089$) for age reflects the fact that the very young are more likely to see a physician than are older children or adults. Males are less likely to initiate a physician contact than females. The significant betas for the three need variables clearly indicate the importance of one's health status in predicting physician contact. People with at least one physician contact tend to be from families having more highly educated heads. Farm residents are less apt to have seen a physician in the year. The lack of a regular source versus having a private doctor for regular care is the strongest predictor of whether or not a physician is seen. Therefore, to increase an individual's possibility of contacting a physician, it is very important to provide them with a regular source of care. The effect of having a hospital ER as regular source of care also has a negative effect on the likelihood of seeing a physician. However, using a hospital OPD for regular care increases one's likelihood of seeing a physician. The lack of insurance is also a significant barrier to a person's initial entry for services.

Employment status has a negative and significant effect, suggesting that the full-time employed are less likely to take time out to see a physician. However, a higher income increases the individual's likelihood of seeing a physician. The shorter length of time in the community predicts a greater likelihood of an initial physician contact. The analysis accounts for 7.4 percent of the variation among people's seeing or not seeing a physician.

The analysis of physician contact for people sixty-five and over (Table 8.12) shows fewer significant predictors, indicating that this group is more homogeneous than those under sixty-five in their physician contact behavior. The direction and magnitudes of those significant predictors are similar to those of people under sixty-five. However, the elderly in the families with unemployed heads or from non-SMSA areas are less likely to have seen a physician. The model accounts for a large proportion (21.5 percent) of variance.

Once the individual has initiated the contact with the physician, their health status becomes the most important predictor of the volume of visits for those under sixty-five, as is evident from the large betas for the three need variables (Table 8.11). This result confirms the findings of previous research that need is even more important for predicting number of visits than for predicting whether or not a physician is seen (Andersen, et al., 1975). Females (beta $= -.027$, $p < .05$) tend to have a greater number of visits. While individuals' volumes of visits do not vary with respect to their poverty level, their numbers of visits may be higher if they are from a family with a more highly educated head or from a high income community. Having public insurance only tends to encourage the individual to visit a doctor more frequently. Finally, the equitable and inequitable variables accounted for 11.3 percent of the variance in people's volume of visits. Table 8.12 shows, that for the elderly sixty-five and over, being female, having poorer perceived health, and using a hospital OPD regularly significantly predict their greater volume of visits.

Hospital Utilization

As can be expected, need has the strongest effect on whether an individual under sixty-five is hospitalized or not (Table 8.11). Perceived health, non-bed disability days, and bed days have strongly significant betas ($p < .001$). Females are much more likely to be admitted to the hospital, which might be a function of admissions for childbirth. Blacks are less apt to be hospitalized than Whites. Having no regular source of care or insurance coverage decreases the individual's likelihood of being hospitalized. However, having both public and private insurance is a positive predictor. The model for hospitalization contributes to 7.8 percent of the variance. Some other inequitable variables (e.g., education and residence) were found not to be significantly correlated with hospitalization and thus were not included in the model.

Among all variables included in the analysis for people sixty-five and over, need variables and sex are the only significant predictors for admissions to the hospital (Table 8.12). Poorer perceived health (beta $= -.093$, $p < .05$) and more non-bed disability days (beta $= .262$, $p < .001$) lead to a greater possibility of being hospitalized. Interestingly, different from those under sixty-five, males as opposed to females over sixty-five are more likely to be admitted to the hospital (beta $= .084$, $p < .05$).

Perceived health (beta $= -.302$, $p < .001$) and non-bed disability days (beta $= .171$, $p < .001$) are the most important predictors of the number of days patients under sixty-five stay in the hospital once admitted. The other significant predictors are age (beta $= .109$, $p < .01$) and sex (beta $= -.161$, $p < .001$). Older adults and females tend to stay in the hospital longer. As can be expected, patients who lack insurance coverage (beta $= -.145$, $p < .001$) tend to stay in the hospital for a shorter period. This is probably due to their inability to pay the costs of longer stays. In contrast, having both public and private insurance to pay for the expenses of hospital stays encourages longer lengths of stay. Having a hospital OPD as a regular source of care also predicts more hospital days. The multiple regression model contributes to a large (28.6 percent) proportion of the variance in the hospital days of those younger than sixty-five.

For those sixty-five and over (Table 8.12), three significant predictors indicate that females and those who have public insurance only tend to stay in the hospital longer but the hospital OPD users stay a shorter length of time once admitted. Non-bed disability days and bed-days are not significant predictors probably because all of the elderly admitted to the hospital have many disability days. Thus, little variance in these two variables results in weak predictive power. It should be noted that, although there are very few significant predictors, the model accounts for a large proportion of the variance (32.7 percent).

Preventive Services

The comparison between three preventive services (blood pressure checks, pap smears, and breast exams) reveals some differences and more similarities. For example, the likelihood of getting the three preventive services is higher among those under sixty-five with higher educational levels. However, poverty level is a significant predictor only for having a blood pressure check among those under sixty-five (beta = .033, $p < .05$). For those under sixty-five, older adults are more likely to have a blood pressure check (beta = .067, $p < .001$); but younger women are more likely to have pap smears and breast exams (See Table 8.11). This may be because hypertension is more of a health risk to older adults while cervical or breast cancer can be more of a risk for younger adults. For those sixty-five and over, however, the older people are less likely to have a blood pressure check. This should be of concern to health professionals. For those under sixty-five, females are more likely than males to have their blood pressure checked, while females sixty-five and over are less likely to do so. For both groups, people with greater needs are more apt to have a blood pressure check. Women under sixty-five who have had a breast exam tend to have better perceived health (beta = .061, $p < .01$) but somewhat more bed days (beta = .046, $p < .05$).

For both age groups not having a regular source of care or insurance coverage are relatively strong predictors; they prevent an individual from obtaining preventive services. For those under sixty-five, using hospital ERs as a regular source of care is also a negative indicator of having a blood pressure check or breast exam. However, the regular hospital OPD users are more likely than private doctor users to have a pap smear or breast exam. For those sixty-five and over, regular hospital OPD users are less likely than private doctor users to have their blood pressure checked.

Ethnicity is not a significant predictor for blood pressure check or breast exam, for those under sixty-five, when other variables are controlled. However, without controlling for other variables (data not shown), Hispanics are somewhat less likely than Whites to have a blood pressure check (beta = -.029, $p < .05$). This is mostly due to their lower educational level, since the magnitude of beta decreases significantly after adjusting for respondents' educational levels. Hispanic women tend to have a pap smear more often than White women (beta = .040, p < .05). For those sixty-five or over, Hispanics are more likely to have a blood pressure check. Without adjusting for other variables (data not shown), Blacks are much less likely than Whites (beta = -.110, p < .001) to have their blood pressure checked. However, the effect becomes insignificant if other variables are held constant. The change of the effect is mostly attributable to the fact that more Blacks use hospital OPDs as their regular source of care, which has a negative impact on having a blood pressure check. Black women are more likely to receive pap smears and breast exams.

Satisfaction

Finally, betas for equitable and inequitable variables regressed on the satisfaction variable show that, for those under sixty-five (see Table 8.11) being younger or a male, new to the community, using hospital OPDs or ERs for regular care or having no regular source of care, or having poorer perceived health and higher non-bed disability days increase an individual's likelihood of not being completely satisfied with a recent physician visit overall. For those over sixty-five, the only significant predictors are poorer perceived health and being White. The elderly who are in ill health or Whites are less likely to be satisfied overall.

Summary

In this chapter, we have described the groups with or without various regular sources of care and insurance coverage with respect to their equitable and inequitable characteristics. In general, the regular private doctor users tend to be a more advantaged group. They are more likely to be Whites from suburban areas and have higher occupational and income levels and private insurance. In contrast, the disadvantaged Blacks tend to name hospital OPDs or other clinics as their regular sources of care. People who report hospital ERs as their regular source of care are more likely to be male and Black. Those who lack a regular source of care are also more likely to have no insurance coverage. They appear to have better health status but have lower educational levels. In terms of insurance coverage for those under sixty-five, while those who have private insurance only are in a higher social class (i.e., higher income, educational or occupational level) and have a lower level of health care needs, the contrary is true for those who have some type of public insurance or no insurance.

We have also examined the differences in medical access between the groups with various regular sources of care and insurance coverage to determine whether the observed differences are attributable to equitable or inequitable variables. The analysis consistently shows that, even with equitable and inequitable variables controlled, those without care or coverage underutilize almost all health services and are more dissatisfied with their most recent visit. Regular hospital ER users also have poorer access to physicians, blood pressure checks, and breast exams. Hospital OPDs appear to provide women who use them regularly better access to pap smears than do other sources of care. Although having public insurance reduces the barriers to physician and hospital services for those who *need* them, it also apparently contributes to some overutilization. This overutilization may be reduced with the constraints being introduced through DRGs and capitated service arrangements for Medicaid-eligible patients.

Finally, we compared the relative importance of equitable and inequitable variables in predicting various access measures. Among all variables included in the analysis, equitable variables, in general, have strongly significant effects on physician and hospital services. Education (of family head or respondent) is an important predictor for physician utilization and preventive services. Most inequitable immutable variables are not related to health services utilization (except physician contact). Lack of a regular source of care or insurance, as expected, uniformly results in poorer access to health services.

As mentioned earlier, all the analyses in this chapter are conducted by using data from the national survey. In the next chapter, we will further explore special access issues by using data available from other studies as well.

Table 8.1. Selection of Regular Source of Care in Relation to Equitable and Inequitable Factors for the U.S. Population (Betas).

CHARACTERISTICS	PRIVATE OFFICE/ CLINIC	HOSPITAL OPD	HOSPITAL ER	OTHER	NO REGULAR SOURCE
EQUITABLE					
Age	-.018	-.012	-.001	-.029*	.060****
Sex	-.087***	.016	.046***	.013	.080****
Need					
Perceived Health	.001	-.057***	-.004	.000	.055****
Non-bed Disability Days	.001	.018	.038***	-.023	-.011
Bed Days	.019	-.015	.017	.013	-.027*
INEQUITABLE-Immutable					
Ethnicity					
Black vs. White	-.093***	.059***	.036**	.049***	.022
Hispanic vs. White	-.007	.004	(.009)	.013	-.006
Other vs. White	-.051***	(.034)	(.016)	(.049)	(-.005)
Education of Head	.009	.022	-.015	.009	-.043**
Occupation of Head	.087***	-.074***	-.006	-.073***	-.002
Poverty Level	.039***	-.009	-.020	-.033*	-.007
Time in Community	.123***	-.053***	-.007	-.054***	-.087***
Per Capita Income	.022	.021	-.017	.039*	.009
M.D.s per 1000 population	-.056***	.020	-.020	.090***	.003
Residence					
Central City vs. Suburb	-.061***	.061***	.012	.015	.023
Non-SMSA vs. Suburb	-.037**	.023	(-.022)	.023	.018
Farm vs. Suburb	-.020	.050***	(-.023)	(.010)	(-.018)
Region					
N. Central vs. East	-.018	-.002	-.011	.038*	.000
West vs. East	-.042**	.019	-.001	.035*	.019
South vs. East	.013	-.033*	-.022	-.012	.021
INEQUITABLE-Mutable					
Insurance Coverage					
Public Only vs. Pvt. Only	-.029*	.043***	(.007)	.016	-.009
Public & Pvt. vs. Pvt. Only	.009	.024	.000	.005	-.038**
None vs. Pvt. Only	-.120***	.063***	.024*	.008	.103***
R^2	.078	.039	.009	.027	.034

* $p < .05$
** $p < .01$
*** $p < .001$
( ) = based on 25 or fewer unweighted cases.

Table 8.2. Selection of Insurance Coverage in Relation to Equitable and Inequitable Factors for the U.S. Population Under 65 and 65 and Over (Betas).

CHARACTERISTICS	PUBLIC ONLY	PRIVATE ONLY	PUBLIC & PRIVATE	NO INSURANCE	PUBLIC ONLY (65 and OVER)
EQUITABLE					
Age	-.017	.015	.028*	-.015	.036
Sex	-.009	.004	.018	-.011	.005
Need					
Perceived Health	-.033*	.062***	-.024	-.036**	-.084*
Non-bed Disability Days	.039**	-.028*	.083***	-.032*	-.058
Bed Days	.093***	-.037**	.004	-.001	.015
INEQUITABLE-Immutable					
Ethnicity					
Black vs. White	.018	.019	.051***	-.059***	.001
Hispanic vs. White	-.011	-.026*	.009	.027*	.141***
Other vs. White	(-.007)	-.024*	(.011)	(.017)	(.063)
Education of Head	-.029*	.038**	-.015	.019	-.036
Occupation of Head	-.076***	.088***	-.061***	-.030*	.021
Poverty Level	-.181***	.316***	-.077***	-.247***	-.178***
Time in Community	-.026*	.017	-.006	.003	-.005
Per Capita Income	.009	-.013	.050	-.034*	-.056
M.D.s per 1000 population	.038*	-.027	.000	.021	.067
Residence					
Central City vs. Suburb	.024	-.051***	.023	.035**	-.014
Non-SMSA vs. Suburb	.008	-.032*	.033*	.012	.038
Farm vs. Suburb	(-.007)	-.003	(-.023)	.016	(.005)
Region					
N. Central vs. East	-.022	.016	.000	-.005	-.061
West vs. East	-.005	-.034*	-.050***	.084***	.062
South vs. East	.056***	.005	-.024	.039*	-.024
INEQUITABLE-Mutable					
Regular Source of Care					
Hospital OPD vs. Pvt. M.D.	.039**	-.067***	-.010	.070***	.040
Hospital ER vs. Pvt. M.D.	(.029)	-.027*	(-.013)	.028*	(-.026)
Other vs. Pvt. M.D.	.016	-.028*	(-.013)	.021	(-.033)
None vs. Pvt. M.D.	(-.021)	-.078***	(-.007)	.111***	.099**
R^2	.093	.192	.039	.114	.110

* $p < .05$
** $p < .01$
*** $p < .001$
( ) = based on 25 or fewer unweighted cases.

Table 8.3.   Percent Seeing a Physician in Last Year, Adjusted for Equitable and Inequitable Factors, According to Regular Source of Care and Insurance Coverage for the U.S. Population.

	UNADJUSTED		ADJUSTED FOR					
			EQUITABLE VARIABLES		INEQUITABLE VARIABLES			
					IMMUTABLE		MUTABLE	
	%	BETA	%	BETA	%	BETA	%	BETA
REGULAR SOURCE OF CARE							Insurance Coverage	
Private Doctor	84	.015	84	.009	84	.012	84	
Hospital OPD	86	.015	85	.009	86	.012	86	.015
Hospital ER	69	-.050***	68	-.053***	69	-.050***	69	-.048***
Other	84	.000	84	.000	84	.002	84	.002
No Regular Source	61	-.187***	62	-.177***	62	-.175***	63	-.166***
INSURANCE COVERAGE							Regular Source of Care	
Less than 65								
Private Only	82		82		82		82	
Public Only	90	.032**	84	.009	86	.015	85	.013
Public & Private	85	.016	83	.005	84	.010	84	.010
No Insurance	70	-.091***	69	-.101***	71	-.086***	73	-.070***
65 and Over								
Public & Private	89		89		89		89	
Public Only	81	-.105**	80	-.123***	81	-.103**	83	-.073*

* p<.05
** p<.01
*** p<.001

Table 8.4.   Mean Visits for Those Seeing a Physician Last Year, Adjusted for Equitable and Inequitable Factors, According to Regular Source of Care and Insurance Coverage for the U.S. Population.

	UNADJUSTED		ADJUSTED FOR					
			EQUITABLE VARIABLES		INEQUITABLE VARIABLES			
					IMMUTABLE		MUTABLE	
	$\bar{X}$	BETA	$\bar{X}$	BETA	$\bar{X}$	BETA	$\bar{X}$	BETA
REGULAR SOURCE OF CARE							Insurance Coverage	
Private Doctor	6.07		6.11		6.13		6.13	
Hospital OPD	7.48	.037**	6.85	.019	6.81	.018	6.77	.017
Hospital ER	6.43	.004	5.12	-.011	5.07	-.012	5.10	-.012
Other	6.44	.009	6.31	.004	6.22	.002	6.18	.001
No Regular Source	4.74	-.036**	5.27	-.023	5.24	-.024	5.28	-.023
INSURANCE COVERAGE							Regular Source of Care	
Less than 65								
Private Only	5.63		5.87		5.88		5.88	
Public Only	12.74	.113***	9.61	.060***	9.54	.058***	9.51	.058***
Public & Private	8.88	.061***	7.12	.023	7.08	.023	7.10	.023
No Insurance	6.32	.019	5.86	.000	5.82	-.001	5.87	.000
65 and Over								
Public & Private	6.68		6.75		6.73		6.74	
Public Only	6.49	-.010	6.22	-.027	6.28	-.023	6.23	-.026

* p < .05
** p < .01
*** p < .001

Table 8.5.   Percent Hospitalized in Last Year, Adjusted for Equitable and Inequitable Factors, According to Regular Source of Care and Insurance Coverage for the U.S. Population.

	UNADJUSTED		EQUITABLE VARIABLES		ADJUSTED FOR INEQUITABLE VARIABLES IMMUTABLE		MUTABLE	
	%	BETA	%	BETA	%	BETA	%	BETA
REGULAR SOURCE OF CARE								Insurance Coverage
Private Doctor	10		10		10		10	
Hospital OPD	12	.017	10	.000	11	.003	11	.004
Hospital ER	15	.018	12	.006	12	.008	12	.009
Other	11	.002	11	.001	11	.004	11	.004
No Regular Source	4	-.063***	6	-.047***	6	-.045***	6	-.039***
INSURANCE COVERAGE								Regular Source of Care
Less than 65								
Private Only	9		9		9		9	
Public Only	20	.061***	12	.016	13	.018	12	.017
Public & Private	17	.055***	13	.023*	13	.026*	13	.026*
No Insurance	6	-.030*	5	-.045***	5	-.044***	5	-.042***
65 and Over								
Public & Private	19		19		19		19	
Public Only	15	-.040	15	-.038	15	-.037	16	-.028

* p<.05
** p<.01
*** p<.001

Table 8.6.   Mean (Logged) Hospital Days for Those Hospitalized in Last Year, Adjusted for Equitable and Inequitable Factors, According to Regular Source of Care and Insurance Coverage for the U.S. Population.

	UNADJUSTED			ADJUSTED FOR EQUITABLE VARIABLES		ADJUSTED FOR INEQUITABLE VARIABLES IMMUTABLE		MUTABLE	
	UNLOGGED X̄	X̄	BETA	X̄	BETA	X̄	BETA	X̄	BETA
REGULAR SOURCE OF CARE								Insurance Coverage	
Private Doctor	9.41	1.69		1.70		1.70		1.69	
Hospital OPD	11.53	1.81	.033	1.65	-.013	1.66	-.012	1.71	.006
Hospital ER	(28.97)	(2.31)	(.091)	(2.18)	(.071)	(2.20)	(.072)	(2.26)	(.083)
Other	9.36	1.49	-.043	1.48	-.049	1.48	-.048	1.49	-.043
No Regular Source	4.86	1.10	-.119**	1.28	-.084*	1.28	-.085*	1.27	-.085*
INSURANCE COVERAGE								Regular Source of Care	
Less than 65									
Private Only	8.89	1.59		1.64		1.63		1.64	
Public Only	10.44	1.81	.050	1.57	-.015	1.63	.002	1.58	-.011
Public & Private	20.56	2.26	.161***	2.03	.095**	2.07	.106**	2.10	.112**
No Insurance	7.74	1.26	-.080*	1.12	-.125***	1.14	-.118**	1.04	-.145***
65 and Over									
Public & Private	9.99	1.79		1.78		1.77		1.78	
Public Only	12.27	2.24	.172*	2.31	.206**	2.35	.225**	2.29	.197**

* p < .05
** p < .01
*** p < .001
( ) = based on 25 or fewer unweighted cases.

Table 8.7.   Percent of Adults 18 and Over Having a Blood Pressure Check, Adjusted for Equitable and Inequitable Factors, According to Regular Source of Care and Insurance Coverage for the U.S. Population.

	UNADJUSTED		ADJUSTED FOR EQUITABLE VARIABLES		ADJUSTED FOR INEQUITABLE VARIABLES IMMUTABLE		MUTABLE	
	%	BETA	%	BETA	%	BETA	%	BETA
REGULAR SOURCE OF CARE							Insurance Coverage	
Private Doctor	82		82		82		82	
Hospital OPD	81	-.007	80	-.011	80	-.008	81	-.005
Hospital ER	64	-.058***	63	-.058***	64	-.055***	64	-.053***
Other	75	-.039**	75	-.035**	76	-.031*	76	-.029*
No Regular Source	56	-.212***	58	-.192***	58	-.187***	59	-.181***
INSURANCE COVERAGE							Regular Source of Care	
Less than 65								
Private Only	78		78		78		77	
Public Only	80	.008	72	-.020	75	-.009	75	-.008
Public & Private	81	.015	78	-.001	79	.005	79	.006
No Insurance	65	-.090***	65	-.094***	67	-.079***	69	-.058***
65 and Over								
Public & Private	87		87		87		87	
Public Only	84	-.037	84	-.042	84	-.036	87	.005

* p<.05
** p<.01
*** p<.001

Table 8.8. Percent of Women 18 and Over Having a Pap Smear, Adjusted for Equitable and Inequitable Factors, According to Regular Source of Care and Insurance Coverage for the U.S. Population.

	UNADJUSTED		ADJUSTED FOR					
			EQUITABLE VARIABLES		INEQUITABLE VARIABLES			
					IMMUTABLE		MUTABLE	
	%	BETA	%	BETA	%	BETA	%	BETA
REGULAR SOURCE OF CARE							Insurance Coverage	
Private Doctor	60		61		61		61	
Hospital OPD	71	.052**	73	.060**	73	.063***	73	.065***
Hospital ER	60	.000	61	.000	60	-.001	61	.000
Other	62	.008	58	-.011	59	-.007	59	-.006
No Regular Source	52	-.052**	48	-.075***	49	-.072***	50	-.064***
INSURANCE COVERAGE							Regular Source of Care	
Less than 65								
Private Only	65		65		64		64	
Public Only	64	-.002	67	.007	71	.021	70	.018
Public & Private	71	.024	75	.042	73	.049	73	.050
No Insurance	50	-.096***	50	-.093***	52	-.079***	53	-.074***
65 and Over								
Public & Private	45		45		45		45	
Public Only	37	-.070	36	-.077	34	-.099	35	-.087

* p<.05
** p<.01
*** p<.001

Table 8.9.   Percent of Women 18 and Over Having a Breast Exam, Adjusted for Equitable and Inequitable Factors, According to Regular Source of Care and Insurance Coverage for the U.S. Population.

| | | | ADJUSTED FOR | | | |
| | UNADJUSTED | | EQUITABLE VARIABLES | | INEQUITABLE VARIABLES IMMUTABLE | | INEQUITABLE VARIABLES MUTABLE |
	%	BETA	%	BETA	%	BETA	%	BETA
REGULAR SOURCE OF CARE							Insurance Coverage	
Private Doctor	68		68		68		68	
Hospital OPD	72	.022	77	.028	74	.033	75	.037
Hospital ER	31#	-.082***	30	-.085***	30	-.084***	30	-.082***
Other	68	.001	66	-.008	67	-.003	67	.000
No Regular Source	48	-.122***	46	-.136***	47	-.130***	48	-.119**
INSURANCE COVERAGE							Regular Source of Care	
Less than 65								
Private Only	69		69		69		69	
Public Only	61	-.029	63	-.022	64	-.008	65	-.012
Public & Private	70	.000	73	.016	74	.023	70	.023
No Insurance	49	-.136***	49	-.130***	51	-.115***	53	-.102***
65 and Over								
Public & Private	63		63		63		62	
Public Only	46	-.147**	46	-.151**	47	-.143**	50	-.109**

* p<.05
** p<.01
*** p<.001
# Differs from Table 7.5. due to missing values on independent variables.

Table 8.10. Percent Not Completely Satisfied Overall with Most Recent Visit, Adjusted for Equitable and Inequitable Factors, According to Regular Source of Care and Insurance Coverage for the U.S. Population.

	UNADJUSTED		ADJUSTED FOR					
			EQUITABLE VARIABLES		INEQUITABLE VARIABLES			
					IMMUTABLE		MUTABLE	
	%	BETA	%	BETA	%	BETA	%	BETA
REGULAR SOURCE OF CARE							Insurance Coverage	
Private Doctor	20		20		21		21	
Hospital OPD	30	.059***	28	.051***	28	.045**	28	.044**
Hospital ER	43	.061***	41	.055***	41	.054***	40	.052***
Other	21	.006	20	.000	19	-.007	20	-.005
No Regular Source	37	.103***	37	.102***	35	.093***	35	.089***
INSURANCE COVERAGE							Regular Source of Care	
Less than 65								
Private Only	23		23		23		24	
Public Only	26	.013	23	.000	21	-.009	20	-.012
Public & Private	22	-.006	19	-.017	18	-.023	18	-.025
No Insurance	32	.060***	31	.050***	30	.044**	28	.031*
65 and Over								
Public & Private	12		12		12		12	
Public Only	15	.041	13	.011	14	.029	14	.028

* p<.05
** p<.01
*** p<.001

Table 8.11.   Relative Importance of Equitable and Inequitable Variables to Access for the U.S. Population Under 65 (Betas).

CHARACTERISTICS	M.D. CONTACT	M.D. VISITS	HOSPITAL-IZATION	HOSPITAL DAYS	B.P. CHECK	PAP SMEAR	BREAST EXAM	SATIS-FACTION
EQUITABLE								
Age	-.089***	-.008	-.007	.109**	.067***	-.152***	-.081***	-.051**
Sex	-.084***	-.027*	-.056***	-.161***	-.062***	-	-	.037***
Need								
Perceived Health	-.059***	-.122***	-.102***	-.302***	-.024	.041	.061**	-.066***
Non-bed Disability Days	.068***	.153***	.145***	.171***	.056***	-.003	.012	.032*
Bed Days	.037**	.166***	.109***	.042	.047**	.030	.046*	.019
INEQUITABLE-Immutable								
Ethnicity								
Black vs. White	.011	-.010	-.037**	.006	.015	.004	.010	.028
Hispanic vs. White	-.004	.016	-.009	.021	-.019	.040*	.005	.026
Other vs. White	-.010	.023	-.011	.017	-.006	.004	-.005	-.007
Education of Head	.076***	.038***	-	-	-	-	-	-
Education of Respondent	-	-	-	-	.043**	.091***	.114***	-
Employment of Head	-.035**	-	-	-	-	-	-	-
Poverty Level	.039**	-.025	-.002	.057	.033*	.024	.009	-.014
Time in Community	-.029*	-	-	-	-	-	-	-.072***
Per Capita Income	-	.034*	-	-	-	-	-	-
Residence								
Central City vs. Suburb	-.008	-	-	-	-	-	-	-
Non-SMSA vs. Suburb	-.025	-	-	-	-	-	-	-
Farm vs. Suburb	-.052***	-	-	-	-	-	-	-
INEQUITABLE-Mutable								
Regular Source of Care								
Hosp. OPD vs. Pvt. M.D.	.025*	.005	.015	.087*	.009	.065**	.048*	.046**
Hosp. ER vs. Pvt. M.D.	-.038**	-.007	.005	(.081)	-.049***	.002	-.084***	.053***
Other vs. Pvt. M.D.	-.004	-.002	-.013	-.054	-.029*	-.012	-.006	.002
None vs. Pvt. M.D.	-.147***	-.022	-.037***	-.037	-.157***	-.056**	-.104***	.095***
Insurance Coverage								
Public Only vs. Pvt. Only	.013	.058***	.017	-.011	-.008	.018	.012	-.012
Public & Pvt. vs. Pvt. Only	.010	.023	.026*	.112**	.006	.050*	.023	-.025
None vs. Pvt. Only	-.070***	.000	-.042***	-.145***	-.058***	-.074***	-.102***	.031*
R^2	.074	.113	.078	.286	.062	.060	.068	.037

* $p < .05$
** $p < .01$
*** $p < .001$
"-" = variable was not used in the analysis.
( ) = based on 25 or fewer unweighted cases.

Table 8.12.   Relative Importance of Equitable and Inequitable Variables to Access for the U.S. Population 65 and Over (Betas).

CHARACTERISTICS	M.D. CONTACT	M.D. VISITS	HOSPITAL-IZATION	HOSPITAL DAYS	B.P. CHECK	PAP SMEAR	BREAST EXAM	SATIS-FACTION
EQUITABLE								
Age	.058	.009	.042	-.051	-.094**	-.168***	-.085	.054
Sex	-.002	-.099**	.084*	-.225**	.068*	—	—	-.014
Need								
Perceived Health	-.167***	-.135**	-.093*	-.133	-.081*	.000	-.026	-.261***
Non-bed Disability Days	.086*	.053	.262***	.109	.107***	.011	.058	.079
Bed Days	.023	.073	.036	.072	.038	.056	.045	-.069
INEQUITABLE-Immutable								
Ethnicity								
Black vs. White	.008	-.002	-.018	(.023)	-.063	.150**	.119*	-.087*
Hispanic vs. White	-.010	.011	-.028	(-.004)	.071*	.089	.045	-.065
Other vs. White	(-.003)	(.004)	(-.018)	—	(-.008)	—	(.027)	(-.009)
Education of Head	.102**	-.028	—	—	.056	.084	.101	—
Education of Respondent	—	—	—	—	—	—	—	—
Employment of Head	.095**	.018	-.041	.069	.028	.028	.088	.033
Poverty Level	.026	.054	—	—	—	—	—	—
Time in Community	-.079*	—	—	—	—	—	—	—
Per Capita Income	—	—	—	—	—	—	—	—
Residence								
Central City vs. Suburb	-.006	—	—	—	—	—	—	—
Non-SMSA vs. Suburb	-.088*	—	—	—	—	—	—	—
Farm vs. Suburb	-.033	—	—	—	—	—	—	—
INEQUITABLE-Mutable								
Regular Source of Care								
Hosp. OPD vs. Pvt. M.D.	-.055	.119**	.050	-.221**	-.095**	.073	-.008	.058
Hosp. ER vs. Pvt. M.D.	(-.119)	(-.028)	(.040)	(.150)	(-.058)	(-.021)	(-.053)	(.008)
Other vs. Pvt. M.D.	-.002	-.007	-.059	(.047)	-.053	(-.036)	(-.033)	-.055
None vs. Pvt. M.D.	-.325***	-.008	-.045	(-.297)	-.377***	-.100*	-.203***	(-.005)
Insurance Coverage								
Public Only vs. Public and Private	-.073*	-.026	-.028	.197**	.005	-.087	-.109*	.028
R^2	.215	.066	.123	.327	.195	.097	.110	.101

* p<.05
** p<.01
*** p<.001
"-" = variable was not used in the analysis.
( ) = based on 25 or fewer unweighted cases.

Chapter 9
Care and Coverage Lessons from the Special Samples

Ronald M. Andersen
Christopher S. Lyttle

T HIS CHAPTER ADDRESSES some questions about the relationship of regular sources of care and financing to access, which one or more of the special studies are especially suited to inform. All of the previous chapters have relied primarily on the national survey while using the special studies to validate, extend or qualify the findings. Because of the unique characteristics of the samples or the information collected in the special studies they can also be used to investigate additional questions including: (1) What is the access to care of low-income people living in states with different Medicaid coverage? (2) Does access differ among Hispanics of Mexican and Puerto Rican origin and Blacks living in different communities? (3) How does access differ for people using innovative forms of ambulatory care compared to those using more traditional sources? and (4) Do health care expenditure patterns vary among people using traditional versus innovative sources of care regularly?

We will focus on physician visits, hospital stays, and satisfaction with recent visits as measures of access. Expenditure measures include those for hospital inpatient care, outpatient department (OPD) and emergency room (ER) visits, physician office visits, as well as total expenditures for medical care. The hierarchical regression model employed in Chapter 8 will also be used here to successively control in the analyses for the effect of: (1) equitable variables — perceived health, disability days, age, and sex; (2) inequitable immutable variables — ethnicity, education of family head, length of residence in community, family size, and family income; and (3) inequitable-mutable variables — insurance coverage and regular source of care. Of special interest will be the importance of both insurance and source of care to the access of the low-income and ethnic samples and the importance of insurance to the access and expenditures of people with innovative versus traditional regular sources of care.

The analytical approach in Chapter 9 differs from earlier chapters in the way the samples are either combined or, in other instances, separated for the various analyses. The low-income samples from NYC, Arizona, and the U. S. are combined in the regression analyses to examine the effect of differential Medicaid coverage on the poor (Table 9.2). Combining is possible because of the common origin of the studies and efforts to construct the variables in a similar fashion (see Chapter 3). Combining samples allows us to compare their access controlling for other differences that might influence access. This allows the comparison of the percent seeing a doctor in NYC and Arizona with the national sample controlling for other potentially important differences such as health status, age, and sex. Similar combining strategies are employed in the analyses of Hispanics and Blacks for which samples from the NYC, Arizona, Community Hospital Program (CHP), Municipal Health Services Program (MHSP), and the U. S. are pooled. Although it is theoretically possible that the same individuals will appear in the community, state, and/or U. S. samples, the actual probability is extremely small. When samples are pooled the sample weights are adjusted so that the sums of the weights for all subsamples are equal. For example, in Table 9.2 the sums of the weights for NYC, Arizona, and the U. S. are all the same, so that we can examine the impact of living one place or another controlling for differences in sample size across the studies.

In other analyses in this chapter samples are separated which have been combined in earlier chapters. This is done when a subsample has characteristics of special interest in an access or expenditure analysis. Thus, in Table 9.2 only the low-income portion of the national sample is included. In the analyses of Hispanic and Black access to care, particular communities from the overall CHP and MHSP samples with significant numbers of ethnic residents have been examined separately. Analyses are then carried out on the ethnic residents of these communities. For example, in Table 9.3 enough Hispanics were found to study separately in the Paterson and Hollywood samples of the CHP study and in the Milwaukee and San Jose samples in MHSP. Finally, the original NYC sample included a probability sample of the entire metropolitan area in addition to a specially screened low-income sample. Other chapters use the total sample while this one is limited to the low-income oversample.

One subsample is included in the analyses in this chapter that has not been considered in previous chapters. It is the sample of persons from the CHP study who have used a CHP site as a source for care, which is referred to in the analyses of access in innovative vs. traditional regular sources of care (Table 9.8). This special sample of patients was drawn from lists provided by the CHP sites and is not included in other CHP analyses in this report, which are based on samples of community residents in the CHP group service areas.

Access of the Poor Under Different State Systems

Medicaid coverage of the poor varies widely from state to state. The comprehensiveness of this coverage might have significant impacts on the health services received by the low-income populations in the respective states. The samples included in this study allow us to examine this important issue.

New York State traditionally has one of the most comprehensive Medicaid programs in terms of both liberal eligibility rules and the scope of services included in the program. In addition, New York City has a large system of public hospitals and associated outpatient clinics dedicated to the treatment of low-income persons. In contrast, Arizona had no Medicaid program at the time this survey was carried out. Individual counties in Arizona had responsibility for providing care to the medically indigent. Eligibility criteria for these county programs were often quite stringent.

Samples from the low-income populations of New York City and the state of Arizona and a comparison sample of the low-income population from the national sample provide a basis for comparing access of the poor under widely varying systems. All sample persons are included from the Arizona sample, since it was a special low-income sample. The criterion for NYC and the national samples was a family income 150 percent of the national poverty level. This criterion seemed preferable to the poverty level since the near poor often have a more difficult time than those below the poverty level because they are not eligible for or shun public programs.

Table 9.1 shows the predisposing, enabling, and need characteristics of each sample. We first examine the equitable variables (age, sex, and health status) because they represent "acceptable reasons" for differences in access according to our definition of equity. Next we follow the social and economic characteristics which are "unacceptable reasons" for variations in access but do not readily suggest directions for health policy to take to alleviate — inequitable-immutable variables. The final set of variables are the key variables in the study — insurance coverage and regular care. They are called inequitable-mutable variables because while they are unacceptable reasons for variation in access they do point the way to policies and programs that might be manipulated to reduce or eliminate this variation.

Table 9.1 shows similar equitable characteristics for NYC and Arizona, with the exceptions that the Arizona sample reports more non-bed disability days and the mean age of the NYC poor is slightly higher. Compared to the U. S. both the special samples report poorer health, are slightly younger, and had more illness requiring them to be in bed all or part of the day.

Both of the special samples have larger proportions of minorities than does the national poverty population as a whole. Sixty percent of the Arizona sample are Hispanic. The other immutable variables show the Arizona sample to be the most disadvantaged. They have less income and education. They are also more transient and have larger families than either the NYC or national poor as a whole.

The Arizona sample also appears to be more disadvantaged than NYC or the national with respect to having insurance coverage or a regular source of care. A larger proportion of the Arizona sample are without insurance (31 percent) or a regular source of care (15 percent). Arizona also has a larger proportion reporting a hospital outpatient department (OPD) as a source of care (29 percent). At the time of this survey Arizona relied on county sources to provide care to the medically indigent. NYC differed from the national poor as a whole in relying more on public coverage than private insurance and more on the hospital than the doctor's office as a source of care. As mentioned earlier, NYC has a relatively generous Medicaid program and an extensive public hospital system.

Table 9.2 concerns various access measures for the NYC, Arizona and U. S. low-income samples. The NYC sample is more likely to see the doctor (79 percent) than the Arizona sample (62 percent). The adjustments for the equitable and inequitable factors make little difference in these comparisons. The behavior of the NYC low-income sample with respect to seeing a doctor is similar to the national low-income sample. Thus, it appears that the Arizona system limited access to physicians for low-income people more so than the NYC approach or the conditions faced by low-income people in the aggregate in the United States.

The number of visits for people seeing the doctor at least once provides a different picture (Table 9.2). The mean number of visits is higher for the Arizona sample (7.40) than for the New York sample (5.74). In this case, the Arizona sample is similar to the nation as a whole (7.38) in numbers of visits received. One possible reason for the excess visits in Arizona compared to NYC is that low-income people wait longer to seek care in Arizona and, consequently, have more serious conditions requiring more visits when they do seek care. It is also correspondingly possible that the more comprehensive system of care in NYC encourages the poor to seek care before they become seriously ill, thus limiting the number of return visits needed.

The percent hospitalized is the same in NYC and Arizona (10%). Both special samples appear less likely to be hospitalized than the national low-income sample. Again, adjustments do not affect the comparisons. The different systems do not appear to markedly influence the admission rates of low-income persons.

The percent not completely satisfied with their last visit to a physician is also similar for NYC (28 percent) and Arizona (29 percent) and not significantly different from the national rate (25 percent). The rates remain similar after adjustment.

In sum, poor people in NYC, which has a wider array of publicly supported care and coverage alternatives, appeared to have greater access to medical care as measured by the proportion seeing the doctor than was true in Arizona. In contrast, the Arizona patients who did see the doctor had more visits, suggesting that once entry is gained, their service needs may be greater. Both the Arizona and NYC poor were less likely to be admitted to a hospital than the national low-income sample, though the level of satisfaction with care was similar across all three samples.

Access of Minorities

Several of the special samples include large proportions of Hispanics or Blacks. We will examine the homogeneity of access patterns among Hispanics and Blacks. Similarities might be expected because of the cultural, social, and economic factors that bind people of the same ethnic groups together. Differences can also be expected because of the pluralism within these groups and the special characteristics of the communities in which they live.

In the analysis of both Hispanic and Black communities the major question is what kind of variation is there within these ethnic groups according to equitable and inequitable characteristics and access to care? Table 9.3 shows the communities from our various samples providing enough respondents of Hispanic origin for special analysis. Two are predominantly Puerto Rican (NYC and Paterson), while four are largely Mexican-American (Arizona, Milwaukee, San Jose, and Hollywood). The national Hispanic sample includes Mexicans, Puerto Ricans, and other Hispanics roughly proportional to their percent in the U.S. population. The samples in Paterson, Milwaukee, San Jose, and Hollywood are not representative of all Hispanics in the respective cities but of the neighborhoods served by a particular CHP or MHSP ambulatory care center. The size of these neighborhoods varied from 117,000 in Milwaukee to 629,000 in Hollywood.

The Hispanics in Arizona report the poorest health and more bed days than other Hispanic samples (Table 9.3). The Arizona and NYC Hispanic samples have relatively more women. The mean age in all the Hispanic communities is less than for the national Hispanic sample and most (except Milwaukee) report more bed disability days.

Arizona Hispanics also appear to be the most economically disadvantaged. They, along with Paterson Hispanics, are least likely to have a high school education, have by far the lowest mean income, and the largest average family size (Table 9.3). All of the communities have lower mean family incomes than the national Hispanic sample.

Insurance coverage and regular source of care differ greatly among these Hispanic samples (Table 9.3). Almost one-half of the Hollywood Hispanics and more than one-third of Arizona report having no insurance coverage. In contrast, only 6 percent in Paterson and 10 percent in Milwaukee report having none. Public only coverage varies from 38 percent in Paterson to 6 percent for the national Hispanic sample, with all communities reporting more public coverage than the national sample. This in part reflects the better socio-economic status in the total national Hispanic sample. While all the communities report less private coverage than the national sample there is great variation among communities — from two-thirds in Milwaukee and San Jose to one-third in Arizona.

The Hollywood Hispanic community is also most likely to be without a regular source of care (40 percent) — twice the rate of any other community examined here. Hispanics are twice as likely to report a doctor's office as a regular source of care in Paterson (73 percent) as they are in Arizona (35 percent). Use of hospital OPDs also differs greatly, ranging from 31 percent in Arizona to 5 percent in Milwaukee.

The data in Table 9.3 have confirmed considerable heterogeneity in the equitable and inequitable characteristics of different Hispanic communities. In Table 9.4 we examine variation in access in these communities as well.

The Puerto Rican communities are more likely to see a doctor than are the Mexican communities (Table 9.4). Adjusting for health status, age, and sex does not change this finding. Further, adjustment for the immutable education and income factors increases the percent seeing a doctor in Arizona (55 to 58 percent). This occurs because Arizona Hispanics have low incomes and educational levels. If these were raised to the national average, use of physicians among Arizona Hispanics is predicted to rise. The final adjustments for insurance coverage and regular source of care show a reduction in Paterson (80 to 74 percent) and an increase in Hollywood (58 to 67 percent) in the proportion seeing a doctor. Paterson had a small proportion (6 percent) without insurance coverage and a large proportion with public coverage (38 percent). The adjustment suggests that if more were without insurance and less with public insurance, access would decline. Hollywood had large portions of Hispanics uninsured and without a regular source of care. The corollary adjustment suggests that if insurance and a regular source were provided to more Hispanics there, the portion seeing a physician would increase.

After all adjustments are completed, it still appears that Puerto Ricans are generally more likely to see a doctor than Mexicans — at least in the communities studied here. The Puerto Rican communities were more like the national sample of Hispanics in the proportion seeing a doctor than were the Mexican communities.

Table 9.4 also shows that the mean number of visits for people seeing the doctor was generally less in the Mexican communities than in the national sample. For the Puerto Rican communities, NYC was lower while Paterson was higher than the national average. The adjustments for demographics and illness show a considerable decline in mean number of visits in Arizona and a substantial increase in Hollywood.* This is not unexpected since Arizona showed the poorest health and Hollywood considerably better. If Arizona Hispanics were in better health, patients would have fewer visits while poorer health would increase the visits in Hollywood.

The adjustments in mean number of visits for inequitable variables show the largest reduction in Paterson and the largest increase in Hollywood (Table 9.4). Paterson showed relatively large proportions of Hispanics with public insurance and a private doctor. The adjustments suggest that Paterson Hispanics' use of private doctors and public insurance coverage accounts for some of their higher utilization. Conversely, it appears that if more Hispanics in Hollywood had insurance and a regular source of care, their mean number of visits would increase.

Table 9.4 shows that the percent of Hispanics hospitalized in four of the six special samples does not differ significantly from the proportion for the U. S. sample (9 percent). Further adjustments do not alter the conclusion for those sites. However, Mil-

---

*Paterson also showed a substantial decline. We attribute this to the outlier cases described in the footnote to Table 9.3.

waukee has a higher rate of hospitalization (14 to 15 percent), and the adjustments do not alter this conclusion either. Conversely, Hollywood has a low unadjusted admission rate (5 percent).* Adjustment for illness raises the proportion to 7 percent, which is not significantly different from the national comparison group. Again this adjustment may reflect the relatively better health reported by Hispanics in Hollywood.

Satisfaction with the last physician visit also varies a great deal across Hispanic communities. Most sites appear less satisfied than the national sample except for New York. However, three appear much more dissatisfied than the rest — Paterson, San Jose, and Hollywood. The adjustments for equitable and inequitable characteristics do not alter these general conclusions.

Table 9.5 shifts the focus to heterogeneity among Black populations. The NYC sample as well as two CHP communities (Paterson and Baltimore) and two MHSP communities (Cincinnati and St. Louis) provided sufficient Black respondents for analysis.

There is considerable variation in equitable and inequitable characteristics among Black as well as Hispanic communities. The portion in fair or poor health varies from 16 percent in Cincinnati to 26 percent in Baltimore (Table 9.5). More than one half are female in each sample but the portion reaches two-thirds in Paterson. The mean age ranges from twenty-three in St. Louis to thirty-two in Baltimore. There is also considerable diversity in disability days with Baltimore having the highest total.

There are important differences in the inequitable immutable variables (Table 9.5). In general, Paterson, Baltimore, and St. Louis Blacks have lower education and income levels and larger families, than NYC and Cincinnati. The latter sites are more similar to the national black sample in these respects.

Similar clusters appear for insurance coverage. Paterson, Baltimore, and St. Louis have relatively more Blacks reporting public only coverage while Blacks in NYC and Cincinnati report more private only coverage. The latter two again look more like the national sample. Most of the special samples are similar to each

---

*It should be noted that Milwaukee and Hollywood are the smallest samples in the Hispanic comparisons and sample size may contribute to the extreme estimates in these sites.

other and slightly higher than the national average (11 percent) in the proportion reporting no insurance (13 to 14 percent).

While Paterson appears relatively disadvantaged, e.g., low income, it has the highest proportion of Blacks reporting a private doctor as a regular source of care (70 percent). One third of the sample in Baltimore and St. Louis report a hospital OPD as a regular source of care and another 18 percent in St. Louis use an ER. More than one fifth of the Cincinnati respondents have some other government or community clinic as a regular source of care. Eleven to 15 percent of the various samples report no regular source of care, with the national sample in between (13 percent).

Turning to access measures, all of the samples except New York show fewer Blacks seeing the doctor than the national average (82 percent) (Table 9.6). St. Louis appears especially low at 66 percent. The adjustments do not change the basic findings. However, the final adjustments suggest that use of private doctors as regular sources of care increased the proportion seeing a doctor in Paterson while regular use of hospital facilities limited the proportion receiving care in St. Louis.

The unadjusted estimates show three of the sites with significantly fewer visits per person than for Blacks in the U. S. sample. Among the special samples, St. Louis has the lowest mean number of visits (4.76) and Baltimore the highest (6.94). The adjustments leave Cincinnati and St. Louis with significantly fewer visits than the U. S.. The most important adjustments are for demographics and illness, showing the sensitivity of number of visits to these measures.

There is considerable variance in hospital use among the black samples. The highest unadjusted rates are found in Baltimore and St. Louis (13 percent). These are relatively low-income black samples relying heavily on public insurance and hospitals for a regular source of care. Paterson has the lowest unadjusted rate (7 percent), is the lowest income sample and relies even more heavily on public insurance. Thus, income and public insurance coverage cannot account for the differences observed. However, the black sample in Paterson is much more likely to have a private doctor as a regular source of care. When adjustments are made for sources of care, the differences between these samples are reduced (up to 9 percent in Paterson and down to 12 percent and 11 percent in Baltimore and St. Louis).

Satisfaction with care shows great variation across the Black samples. Paterson and Baltimore Blacks are relatively dissatisfied (37 and 45 percent are not completely satisfied). Conversely, Cincinnati and St. Louis report only 23 percent not completely satisfied. The adjustments show that most of this variation cannot be explained with the control variables. However, the final adjustment for mutable variables does show Blacks in Paterson would be even more dissatisfied if fewer of them used a private doctor. In contrast, Blacks in Baltimore and St. Louis might be less dissatisfied if they relied less on hospital OPDs.

These analyses of access for special samples of Hispanics and blacks have pointed out wide variations within major ethnic groups depending on location and other equitable and inequitable factors. Insurance coverage and regular source of care, for example, certainly play an important role in the care and satisfaction with services of Hispanics and Blacks. However, the nature of that role may vary considerably among communities, depending on the dominant systems of care and coverage available.

Access in Innovative Ambulatory Models

Up to this point our analysis has focused on access as a function of more "traditional" sources of care including doctors' offices, hospital OPDs and ERs, and not having a regular source of care. For the past two decades a number of alternative forms of ambulatory care have emerged as important, or potentially important, regular sources of care. In addition to the growth of HMOs, new forms include independent practice associations, preferred provider organizations, emergicenters, and a plethora of primary care centers with various combinations of sponsorship and financing. While we have neither the data nor resources to examine all of these alternative forms in detail, our special CHP and MHSP samples do allow us to explore two versions of primary care centers and compare their impact on access with the impact of traditional forms of regular care.

The Community Hospital Program (CHP) was developed by the Robert Wood Johnson Foundation in the early 1970s to promote access to primary care for patients and their families on a continuing basis. Community hospitals were to offer patients a primary care group practice, with full time professional staff and appropriate technical support. The group practices were to be co-sponsored by the hospital medical staff to facilitate integration of primary, secondary, and tertiary services. Fifty-three hospitals were given up to $500,000 each for four years of planning and development. The groups were staffed predominantly by family practitioners and internists. A third of the groups used nonphysician providers, usually nurse practitioners. Eleven CHP sites were included in our sample to represent a cross-section of the hospitals and communities included in the overall program (Aday, et. al., 1985; Shortell, et. al. 1984).

The Municipal Health Services Program (MHSP) was similar to the CHP in promoting primary care centers intended to provide continuous care and improve community access to needed services. It was launched by the Robert Wood Johnson Foundation in 1977 with an invitation to the fifty largest cities in the United States to submit proposals for a network of three or more clinics located apart from public hospital campuses in neighborhoods of documented need. Five cities (Baltimore, Cincinnati, Milwaukee, St. Louis, and San Jose) were awarded grants of up to three million dollars for planning and partial support of service delivery. The Health Care Financing Administration joined the project, offering Medicare and later Medicaid waivers to the funded clinics. The waivers included elimination of coinsurance and deductibles for Medicare and coverage for a range of additional services, if offered at the clinics, including dental, prescribed drugs, optometry and podiatry services. In each of the five cities one clinic was chosen for the evaluation based on the ability to clearly define a service area and the expectation that the clinic might have a measurable impact on access to care (Fleming and Andersen, 1986).

In the following analyses we will then compare people who use the CHP or MHSP program as their regular source of care with other people in the communities where the clinics are located who use the traditional sources of regular care analyzed throughout this study. For each program attention will focus first on whether the characteristics of people served by these programs differ from others in the community and then on differences in access between the users of the special programs and people with other regular sources of care. Observations in the CHP analyses are unweighted because we are combining samples of patients from the CHP clinics with those from community surveys in all eleven sites and appropriate weights are not available. The analysis is appropriate for examining relationships among variables although we are unable to accurately estimate parameters of known populations. The MHSP analyses, however, are based on weighted observations which are probability samples of the service areas of the MHSP clinics.

Table 9.7 shows that persons who consider CHP clinics to be their regular source of care have equitable and inequitable characteristics most similar to regular users of private physicians. They have similar health and gender distributions although CHP patients are younger (29.0 vs. 33.2 mean years of age). CHP patients appear in better health than those who use OPDs and not so different from ER and other clinic regular users. They are, however, in poorer health than people without a regular source of care.

CHP patients are also quite similar to users of private doctors with respect to inequitable-immutable factors (Table 9.7)— including ethnicity, work status, education, and income. CHP users do appear to have lived in their current neighborhood less time than private doctor users. They are less likely to be minority and have higher income and education levels than users of other sources of care (excluding users of private doctors). CHP users appear more mobile than hospital (OPD or ER) users but less so than people using other clinics or having no regular care.

To complete this picture of CHP users' similarity to private doctor users, their health insurance coverage looks the same (Table 9.7). Compared to other types of users, CHP users are generally more likely to have private and less likely to have public insurance coverage.

Table 9.8 suggests relatively high access of CHP users in use of physicians and satisfaction and lower inpatient hospital utilization. Estimates of the percent seeing a doctor are as high or higher for CHP users as for private doctor, hospital OPD, and other clinic users—both unadjusted and adjusted for other characteristics. The proportion of CHP users seeing a doctor is much higher than the proportion for ER users and those without a regular source of care.

While Table 9.8 shows no significant differences between mean number of physician visits for CHP users and other users, some of the substantive differences are still worth noting. The unadjusted estimates show CHP and private doctor users to be very similar. In contrast, the mean number of visits for hospital users and patients in other clinics appear higher while the estimate for those without a regular source appears lower. The adjustment for health (equitable factors) decreases the estimate for OPD users and increases the estimate for those without a regular source of care. These results suggest that if OPD users had better health and those without a regular source were less healthy, the number of visits they receive in a year when they seek care might be quite similar to the number for CHP users. The adjustments do not change the estimates much for ER users, suggesting that while they are less likely to seek care than CHP patients, once they do, they may have more visits regardless of their health status.

One purpose of the CHP program was to de-emphasize inpatient hospital services while concentrating on primary ambulatory care services. The data in Table 9.8 evidence some success in the program's attaining this objective. OPD users are significantly more likely to be admitted to a hospital than are CHP users (19 vs. 10 percent) according to the unadjusted estimates. The adjustment reduces the difference (15 vs. 10 percent), but it is still significant. Private doctor, ER and other clinic users appear somewhat more likely to be admitted to a hospital than CHP users although the differences are not significant. Still, the differences remain after all adjustments. Only those without a regular source of care appear less likely to be admitted to a hospital than CHP users. Even those differences become statistically insignificant once we control for the better health of those without a regular source of care.

CHP users appear much more satisfied than users of all other sources except private doctors (Table 9.8). This is true for the adjusted as well as unadjusted estimates. Private doctor users appear slightly less satisfied than CHP users but the results are not statistically significant.

Table 9.9 suggests that the MHSP attracted regular users from the communities they served that differed considerably from those attracted by the CHP program. Compared to users of other regular care sources MHSP users were relatively young and in good health. They include large proportions of minorities, less educated and low-income individuals. They also rely heavily on public insurance or are uninsured. Thus, while the CHP appeared to attract patients that as a group mirrored many of the characteristics of the larger community, the MHSP seemed to attract people who were in relatively good health but disadvantaged economically.

MHSP patients had a mean age (21.8) several years younger than any comparison group and also had the largest proportion of females (62 percent) (Table 9.9). They also appear to be in better health than any other group except those without any regular source of care.

They are clearly the outlier group when inequitable immutable factors are considered (Table 9.9). Compared to all other groups, ranging from those with a private doctor to those without any regular source of care, regular MHSP users include more minorities and people not working full time. Their mean years of education, income, and years in the city are lowest while their family size is largest.

MHSP patients are most likely to have public coverage (Table 9.9). Also, along with ER users and those without a regular source of care, they are least likely to have any insurance. MHSP then appears to be reaching a group with limited resources for covering their health care costs — disproportionately young, female, minority, unemployed, low-income, and members of large families.

Table 9.10 shows an access pattern for MHSP users not so different from CHP users, even though the kinds of people selected into the two programs are apparently quite different. MHSP (like the CHP) patients show relatively high access to physician services, moderate use of the inpatient services, and higher satisfaction than other groups, excepting those using private doctors.

The percent of MHSP patients seeing the doctor in a year is similar to the proportion for those going to a private doctor. It appears higher than those going to other sources and is much higher than the percent for those without a regular source. The results are not altered much by the adjustments for equitable and inequitable factors.

The number of visits received by persons getting physician care at the MHSP site appears generally higher than for persons with other sources of care (Table 9.10). Only patients using OPDs have as many visits on average and adjustment for their poorer health level drops their average under that of MHSP users, but not significantly.

Regular users of private doctors and hospitals are more likely to be hospitalized than MHSP users (Table 9.10). Again, adjustment for health status reduces the percent for hospital OPD users (from 17 to 15 percent), but the adjusted rate remains significantly higher than that for MHSP users (12 to 11 percent). Other clinic users appear to have lower rates but not significantly. Persons without a regular source of care have considerably lower unadjusted rates (7 percent). Taking into account their better health increases the proportion to 9 percent, which is still significantly less than the MHSP rate.

Finally, the proportion not completely satisfied with their last visit is 31 percent of MHSP users, which is less than for all other comparison groups except users of private doctors (25 percent) (Table 9.10). Adjustment for equitable factors reduces the difference between MHSP (29 percent) and private doctor users (26 percent), though it remains statistically significant.

In this section we have examined the access implications of some innovative forms of ambulatory care. Though the characteristics of MHSP and CHP users were quite different, their access patterns, in generally, compared favorably with users of other sources of care or individuals with no regular provider. In the final section of the chapter we turn to the cost implications of one of these organizational forms: the Municipal Health Services Program (MHSP)

Comparing Expenditures of Persons with MHSP and Other Regular Sources of Care

The innovative ambulatory care forms have implications for expenditures as well as access to needed services. The emphasis on primary, continuous services might lead to increased ambulatory care which could increase costs. Private doctors may be able to provide services even more cheaply than the organized ambulatory care programs. However, increased efforts on prevention, early detection, and control of chronic conditions might reduce expensive serious episodes and the need for hospitalization. Also, providing primary care in an ambulatory setting rather than OPDs or ERs associated with high overhead costs may also reduce expenditures. The MHSP study gathered data allowing us to examine expenditures by persons using the traditional sources of regular care compared to those using the MHSP.

Respondents have difficulty accurately reporting medical care expenditures, particularly hospital expenditures. Earlier work has suggested that fairly reliable expenditure information could be obtained from a careful use of estimation algorithms based on respondent reports of medical care use and insurance coverage and expenditure estimates from external sources (Andersen, et al., 1979). Survey data from respondents reporting out-of-pocket and total hospital expenditures were, therefore, supplemented with information from numerous sources in arriving at our final expenditures estimates. Thus, unit charge estimates were obtained from the American Hospital Association for hospital days and outpatient visits, the National Medical Care Expenditures Survey for physician visits, and Medicare fee schedules for surgical procedures. Unit cost estimates for MHSP services were obtained from administrative reports submitted by the MHSP clinics to the Robert Wood Johnson Foundation (Fleming and Andersen, 1986).

Per capita expenditures for persons with different regular sources of care were estimated using a two-step process (Duan, et al., 1983). First, the probability of having expenditures for different types of services was estimated using the same procedures employed elsewhere in this chapter for estimating the probability of use, e.g., estimating percent seeing an M.D. in Table 9.2. In the second stage, expenditures for those using the service are estimated. The dependent variable is the natural log of the relevant expenditures. The independent variables in the second stage are the same as those employed in the first stage. The logged results are then converted back to dollar units.* Finally, the estimated mean expenditure for people using a service (from stage 2) is multiplied by the estimated percent using it (from stage 1) to get the estimated per capita expenditure.

Significance tests were computed on the probability of having

---

*This process is described in Fleming and Andersen, 1986, drawing on a rationale developed by Miller, 1984. The dollar estimates given here reflect expenditures taking place largely in 1982. They have *not* been adjusted upward for medical care price inflation.

expenses for the various services shown: hospital inpatient, visits to a hospital OPD or ER, other visits to a physician, and all other services including drugs, dental care, and other medical appliances and services. Significance tests were also performed on the volume of expenditure for those people with expenditures. In both instances the comparison is between MHSP patients and people with other regular sources of care. In Table 9.11, the significance of the probability of expenditure and the volume of expenditures are indicated separately. The total expenditures column at the bottom of the table represents the simple sum of the expenditures for all of the services shown.

The unadjusted expenditures for inpatient services show the largest values for people whose regular source of care is a hospital — either OPD ($807) or ER ($744). People with a private doctor as a regular source have the next largest inpatient per capita expenditures ($672). People with another clinic ($503) or the MHSP facility ($457) follow. Those with no source of care have the lowest mean expenditures for the inpatient services ($329).

The controls for health status and age and sex cause a large reduction in the estimates for the OPD users (to $727) — since they report the poorest health status; and a large increase for those with no regular source — since they report the best health status (to $435). Other major adjustments are an increase in the estimate for ER users when adjustments are made for health (because they are a relatively healthy population) and an increase in the estimate for those with no regular source when controlling for health insurance coverage (because they are less likely to have health insurance).

When all the adjustments are made the general ordering remains. The main alterations suggest: (1) ER users' hospital expenditures are adjusted upwards; and (2) people with no regular source of care also have higher estimated expenditures, after adjusting for health and inequitable factors. After adjustment, the MHSP inpatient expenditures tend to increase because the MHSP users are in relatively good health and have low incomes. MHSP users' hospital expenditures, however, continue to appear modest — only $31 per person more than the expenditures for people without a regular source of care.

Per capita expenditures for OPD and ER expenditures are, not unexpectedly, highest for people who use those facilities as their regular source of care. Those using OPDs average $220 per person per year and those using ERs average $156. In contrast, users of all other sources as well as those without a regular source average between $40 and $50 per year. Adjustments do not alter the general magnitude or relationship of expenditures among the various sources of care. MHSP users, then, have much lower OPD and ER expenditures than regular users of hospitals and only slightly higher OPD and ER expenditures than people seeing private doctors.

MHSP patients have the highest unadjusted expenditures for doctor visits ($177) excluding visits to ERs and OPDs (Table 9.11). Regular users of private doctors have the second highest expenditures ($134) with people using other types of clinics third highest ($115). The lowest office visit expenditures are experienced by people without a regular source of care ($56) and regular users of hospitals (ER users–$53; OPD users–$44), whose outpatient expenditures are largely in hospitals. Adjustments for equitable and inequitable factors do not alter the rankings or appreciably change the magnitude of these estimates.

Regular users of private doctors have the highest mean yearly unadjusted expenditures for other medical services including drugs and dental care ($225) (Table 9.11), with users of OPDs ($212) and other clinics ($181) also having relatively high expenditures. In contrast, regular users of ERs ($139) and MHSP clinics ($132) and people without a regular source of care ($135) have considerably lower other expenditures. The adjustments generally increase the estimated expenditures for the groups with the lowest unadjusted values. The largest increases are for the MHSP clinic users. Adjustments for health status and age increase the estimate some ($143), but the biggest increases result from the inequitable immutable variables ($174). The latter increase reflects the low income and education of the MHSP patients, which apparently depresses their use of ancillary services (including dental care and drugs).

Total expenditures vary considerably according to what source people use for their regular care (Table 9.11). Hospital OPDs ($1192) and ERs ($1200) appear to be the most expensive sources even after adjustments for the relatively poor health of the OPD users and for the relatively good health of ER users. The higher total expenses result from *both* large hospital inpatient and hospital outpatient components. Adjusted total expenses for the majority group who use private doctors as a regular source of care are $1026 per year—intermediate among all sources of care. They have relatively high doctor visit and ancillary expenses but more moderate expenses for other categories of service. MHSP users have relatively modest adjusted total expenses ($906) among people with a regular source of care. High physician visit costs are more than compensated for by low inpatient costs for MHSP users. Unadjusted total expenses appear even lower for MHSP users with the largest adjustment upwards being made for inequitable immutable variables (e.g., low income and education). Total adjusted expenses for other clinic users ($879) are most similar to those for MHSP users. Finally, persons without a regular source of care have the lowest adjusted total expense ($728). The unadjusted estimates ($561) are even lower than the adjusted, but this is largely because of the relatively good health status of this group which reduces the demand for services.

Summary

This chapter has examined some questions about access and medical care organization and financing made possible by the diversity of data sets employed in this study. First, we explored how the low-income populations fared under more and less comprehensive state insurance coverage. Under the more comprehensive system (New York City) the low-income population were more likely to see a doctor. The number of visits once a doctor was seen were greater in the less comprehensive system (Arizona). Once entry was gained then the ambulatory service needs of the Arizona poor appeared to be greater. The populations did not differ in the rates of hospitalization or levels of satisfaction with care, however.

Next we addressed differences in access among ethnic groups living in different communities. Large differences were observed, as highlighted by the greater likelihood that Hispanics from largely Puerto Rican neighborhoods were more likely to see a doctor than those from predominantly Mexican neighborhoods. Communities of Blacks also varied considerably across all measures of access including doctor visits, hospitalization rates, and satisfaction. Care and coverage played an important role in predicting access of minorities. However, remaining unexplained differences point up the varying needs among ethnic communities.

The third question concerned relative access for persons in innovative ambulatory care programs compared to persons with more traditional sources of regular care. The two programs considered—the CHP and the MHSP—both seemed to facilitate access to physicians while limiting inpatient use when compared to most other regular sources of care.

Finally, we examined the expenditures for people with different sources of regular care including one innovative program—MHSP. This study suggested that hospital OPDs and ERs were a relatively expensive source of regular care while private doctors' offices and other clinics were somewhat less expensive. The MHSP appeared to contain expenditures by substituting office visits in neighborhood facilities for more expensive inpatient services and ambulatory visits to hospitals.

Table 9.1   Characteristics of Near Poverty Populations.

CHARACTERISTICS	NYC	ARIZONA Low Income	U.S.
EQUITABLE			
Fair or Poor Health	31%	32%	26%
Female	57	58	57
Age (Mean Years)	31.6	30.4	32.8
Disability Days:			
In Bed (Mean)	7.2	7.3	6.1
Other (Mean)	10.0	16.0	16.5
INEQUITABLE-Immutable			
White	32	27	67
Hispanic	42	60	10
Black	23	9	21
Less than High School	41	61	39
0-10 Years in Community	23	50	45
Family Size (Mean)	3.8	4.4	3.7
Family Income (Mean $)	9005	5503	8031
INEQUITABLE-Mutable			
Insurance Coverage			
Public Only	24	25	13
Private Only	42	32	49
Public and Private	14	11	16
None	20	31	22
Regular Source of Care			
Private Office/Clinic	51	38	66
Hospital OPD	21	29	11
Hospital ER	7	2	3
Other Clinic	10	15	8
None	11	15	12
Table n	1040	3655	3502

Table 9.2   Access to Care of Near Poverty Populations.

ACCESS MEASURE	NYC	ARIZONA Low Income	U.S.
Percent Seeing M.D.			
Unadjusted	79	62***	79
Adjusted for:			
Equitable	79	62***	79
Inequitable:			
Immutable	79	64***	77
Mutable	79	64***	77
Mean M.D. Visits			
Unadjusted	5.74***	7.40	7.38
Adjusted for:			
Equitable	5.76***	7.22	7.54
Inequitable:			
Immutable	5.39***	7.65	7.48
Mutable	5.20***	7.68	7.65
Percent Hospitalized			
Unadjusted	10*	10	12
Adjusted for:			
Equitable	10*	10	12
Inequitable:			
Immutable	10	10	12
Mutable	10*	10	12
Percent Not Completely Satisfied Overall			
Unadjusted	28	29	25
Adjusted for:			
Equitable	28	28	26
Inequitable:			
Immutable	29	29	25
Mutable	29	28	26

Significantly different from U.S.:
  * $p < .05$
 ** $p < .01$
*** $p < .001$

Table 9.3   Characteristics of Hispanic Populations.

CHARACTERISTICS	Primarily Puerto Rican		Primarily Mexican				Total U.S.
	NYC	Pater -son	Arizona Low Inc	Milwau -kee	San Jose	Holly -wood	
EQUITABLE							
Fair or Poor Health	24%	21%	34%	17%	24%	18%	18%
Female	57	47	57	47	51	46	50
Age (Mean Years)	27.3	21.5	26.6	25.0	24.0	25.7	28.3
Disability Days:							
In Bed (Mean)	5.1	4.4#	5.6	2.6	4.9	6.0	3.3
Other (Mean)	6.9	6.5	9.5	4.7	8.2	1.6	8.5
INEQUITABLE-Immutable							
Less than High School	49	70	72	52	53	56	26
Family Size (Mean)	3.8	4.1	4.9	4.4	4.5	4.1	4.1
Family Income (Mean $)	14182	10663	5842	19875	20820	13320	22249
INEQUITABLE-Mutable							
Insurance Coverage							
Public Only	23	38	23	22	17	11	6
Private Only	49	56	34	66	64	44	71
Public and Private	5	*	7	1	3	*	6
None	22	6	35	10	16	45	17
Regular Source of Care							
Private Office/Clinic	51	73	35	51	44	40	71
Hospital OPD	19	8	31	5	15	7	8
Hospital ER	7	1	2	2	6	2	2
Other Clinic	11	4	17	21	16	11	7
None	12	13	15	21	19	40	12
Table n	840	148	1959	290	1337	172	563

* less than .5 percent.
# This number excludes five highly weighted outliers. The mean including these cases is 33.2.

Table 9.4   Access to Care of Hispanic Populations.

ACCESS MEASURE	Primarily Puerto Rican		Primarily Mexican				Total U.S.
	NYC	Pater -son	Arizona Low Inc	Milwau -kee	San Jose	Holly -wood	
Percent Seeing M.D.							
Unadjusted	81	79	57***	72***	68***	55***	80
Adjusted for:							
Equitable	80	79	55***	73***	67***	57***	81
Inequitable:							
Immutable	79	80	58***	72**	67***	58***	78
Mutable	77	74	58***	72	68***	67***	76
Mean M.D. Visits							
Unadjusted	5.22**	8.49**	6.66	4.25***	5.16**	4.36***	6.91
Adjusted for:							
Equitable	5.19***	8.14	6.01**	4.45***	4.92***	5.09***	7.25
Inequitable:							
Immutable	4.91***	8.03	6.21	4.59***	5.18***	5.02***	7.11
Mutable	4.75***	7.67	6.28	4.65***	5.17***	5.38***	7.17
Percent Hospitalized							
Unadjusted	8	7	9	14***	8	5**	9
Adjusted for:							
Equitable	7	8	7	15***	8	7	9
Inequitable:							
Immutable	7	8	7	15***	8	7	8
Mutable	6	8	7	15***	8	7	9
Percent Not Completely Satisfied Overall							
Unadjusted	24	48***	30	32*	40***	48***	26
Adjusted for:							
Equitable	24	48***	29	32	39***	49***	27
Inequitable:							
Immutable	24	50***	32**	30**	37***	51***	23
Mutable	24	54***	31*	31*	36***	49***	24

Significantly different from U.S.:
 * p<.05
 ** p<.01
*** p<.001

Table 9.5   Characteristics of Black Populations.

CHARACTERISTICS	NYC	Paterson	Balti-more	Cincin-nati	St. Louis	Total U.S.
EQUITABLE						
Fair or Poor Health	21%	19%	26%	16%	23%	24%
Female	59	67	57	58	62	53
Age (Mean Years)	29.3	25.5	32.2	29.8	23.3	30.5
Disability Days:						
In Bed	7.5	10.4	7.6	3.5	1.9	5.7
Other	7.5	4.9	13.8	15.2	12.5	12.5
INEQUITABLE-Immutable						
Less than High School	25	58	54	27	45	32
Family Size (Mean)	3.7	4.3	4.2	3.9	4.4	3.9
Family Income (Mean $)	17294	9162	12998	18149	11215	17685
INEQUITABLE-Mutable						
Insurance Coverage						
Public Only	12	42	35	17	35	9
Private Only	63	44	44	62	43	67
Public and Private	12	1	7	7	6	13
None	13	13	14	14	17	11
Regular Source of Care						
Private Office/Clinic	50	70	35	51	25	59
Hospital OPD	21	8	33	11	33	14
Hospital ER	6	1	7	6	18	3
Other Clinic	11	10	13	22	9	10
None	11	11	11	10	15	13
Table n	569	167	513	1197	495	688

Table 9.6   Access to Care of Black Populations.

ACCESS MEASURE	NYC	Paterson	Balti-more	Cincin-nati	St. Louis	Total U.S.
Percent Seeing M.D.						
Unadjusted	85	77*	77**	78*	66***	82
Adjusted for:						
Equitable	86	77**	77**	79*	64***	82
Inequitable:						
Immutable	84	78*	78*	78*	65***	82
Mutable	85	75***	78*	77**	68***	82
Mean M.D. Visits						
Unadjusted	5.80*	6.13	6.94	5.29***	4.76***	6.84
Adjusted for:						
Equitable	6.04	6.69	6.55	5.38**	4.41***	6.68
Inequitable:						
Immutable	6.11	6.50	6.52	5.51**	4.30***	6.81
Mutable	6.22	6.41	6.39	5.56***	4.18***	7.01
Percent Hospitalized						
Unadjusted	9	7	13***	10	13***	9
Adjusted for:						
Equitable	10	8	12**	10	12**	8
Inequitable:						
Immutable	10	8	12**	10	12*	8
Mutable	9	9	12**	11*	11**	8
Percent Not Completely Satisfied Overall						
Unadjusted	30	37***	45***	23	23	26
Adjusted for:						
Equitable	30	37***	45***	24	21*	26
Inequitable:						
Immutable	30	37***	45***	24	21*	26
Mutable	30	42***	42***	24	17***	28

Significantly different from U.S.:
  * p<.05
 ** p<.01
*** p<.001

Table 9.7   Characteristics of Persons Using CHP and Other Sites as Their Regular Source of Care in CHP Evaluation.

CHARACTERISTICS	Pvt. M.D.	Hosp. OPD	Hosp. ER	Other Clinic	None	CHP
EQUITABLE						
Fair or Poor Health	17%	32%	22%	22%	11%	16%
Female	56	57	41	57	43	55
Age (Mean Years)	33.2	35.4	30.3	30.0	33.9	29.0
Disability Days:						
In Bed (Mean)	3.4	5.6	2.9	4.1	1.7	3.2
Other (Mean)	14.6	22.1	13.7	10.2	6.7	14.1
INEQUITABLE-Immutable						
White	82	30	62	41	72	81
Hispanic	6	9	5	11	12	6
Black	11	59	33	46	14	12
Not Working Full Time	30	56	38	43	28	28
Less than High School	31	58	44	45	32	31
Years in Neighborhood	13.9	13.7	13.1	11.3	10.1	12.3
Family Size (Mean)	3.5	3.9	3.8	4.0	3.4	3.8
Family Income (Mean $)	20535	11866	14447	15327	18341	20311
INEQUITABLE-Mutable						
Insurance Coverage						
Public Only	14	41	18	36	9	17
Private Only	72	38	59	38	62	69
Public and Private	8	8	6	11	6	6
None	7	13	17	15	23	9
Table n	5342	507	209	225	1082	1832

Table 9.8   Access to Care of CHP and Other Sources of Regular Care in CHP Evaluation.

ACCESS MEASURE	Pvt. M.D.	Hosp. OPD	Hosp. ER	Other Clinic	None	CHP
Percent Seeing M.D.						
Unadjusted	85**	85	67***	85	49***	90
Adjusted for:						
Equitable	85**	82**	68***	84	51***	89
Inequitable:						
Immutable	85**	83*	69***	84	52***	89
Mutable	85**	82*	69***	84	53***	89
Mean M.D. Visits						
Unadjusted	6.20	7.50	7.60	6.88	5.15	6.19
Adjusted for:						
Equitable	6.18	6.09	7.54	6.62	6.06	6.13
Inequitable:						
Immutable	6.22	5.79	7.46	6.38	5.97	6.20
Mutable	6.22	5.68	7.54	6.15	6.08	6.16
Percent Hospitalized						
Unadjusted	12	19***	12	11	6*	10
Adjusted for:						
Equitable	12	15*	12	11	8	10
Inequitable:						
Immutable	12	15*	12	11	8	10
Mutable	12	15*	12	11	9	10
Percent Not Completely Satisfied Overall						
Unadjusted	30	53***	56***	44**	41***	27
Adjusted for:						
Equitable	30	51***	56***	43**	43***	27
Inequitable:						
Immutable	31	48***	55***	41*	41***	27
Mutable	31	48***	55***	41*	41***	27

Significantly different from CHP:
* p<.05
** p<.01
*** p<.001

Table 9.9   Characteristics of Persons Using MHSP and
            Other Sites as Their Regular Source of Care
            in MHSP Evaluation.

CHARACTERISTICS	Pvt. M.D.	Hosp. OPD	Hosp. ER	Other Clinic	None	MHSP
EQUITABLE						
Fair or Poor Health	16%	23%	19%	16%	12%	16%
Female	57	53	47	54	45	62
Age (Mean Years)	33.6	29.1	26.7	26.4	31.7	21.8
Disability Days:						
In Bed (Mean)	4.4	5.5	3.9	3.2	2.7	2.6
Other (Mean)	15.4	21.0	10.5	14.6	7.9	12.9
INEQUITABLE-Immutable						
White	78	55	53	57	65	39
Hispanic	10	16	17	21	21	31
Black	9	23	28	14	10	27
Not Working Full Time	29	40	39	39	30	49
Education (Mean Years)	12.0	11.3	10.9	11.3	11.7	9.8
Years in City (Mean)	30.2	26.0	25.6	22.7	23.9	21.4
Family Size (Mean)	3.4	3.7	3.8	3.9	3.3	4.4
Family Income (Mean $)	22485	18262	18195	17914	19962	10900
INEQUITABLE-Mutable						
Insurance Coverage						
Public Only	13	26	21	25	12	32
Private Only	70	54	52	54	59	37
Public and Private	11	9	5	9	5	9
None	6	11	23	13	25	22
Table n	6987	1572	757	742	1992	1204

Table 9.10   Access to Care of MHSP and Other Sources of Regular Care in MHSP Evaluation.

ACCESS MEASURE	Pvt. M.D.	Hosp. OPD	Hosp. ER	Other Clinic	None	MHSP
Percent Seeing M.D.						
Unadjusted	81	78***	65***	78**	43***	82
Adjusted for:						
Equitable	81	77**	65***	78*	45***	80
Inequitable:						
Immutable	81*	77***	66***	78***	45***	83
Mutable	80**	76***	68***	77***	47***	83
Mean M.D. Visits						
Unadjusted	5.21*	5.83	4.48	5.14*	4.28***	5.70
Adjusted for:						
Equitable	5.15**	5.41	4.53	5.20*	4.77***	5.74
Inequitable:						
Immutable	5.16**	5.43	4.59	5.17*	4.71***	5.84
Mutable	5.15**	5.37	4.62	5.14*	4.79***	5.80
Percent Hospitalized						
Unadjusted	14*	17***	14	10	7***	12
Adjusted for:						
Equitable	14**	15***	14**	10	9**	11
Inequitable:						
Immutable	14*	15***	15*	10	9***	12
Mutable	14*	15**	15**	10	9**	12
Percent Not Completely Satisfied Overall						
Unadjusted	25***	39***	35*	37**	37***	31
Adjusted for:						
Equitable	26*	37***	34**	35***	37***	29
Inequitable:						
Immutable	26**	38***	35**	35*	36***	31
Mutable	26**	38***	35**	35*	36***	30

Significantly different from MHSP:
  * p<.05
 ** p<.01
*** p<.001

Table 9.11   Per Capita Expenditures for Services by
MHSP Patients and Those with Other
Sources of Regular Care in MHSP
Evaluation.

SERVICE	Pvt. M.D.	Hosp. OPD	Hosp. ER	Other Clinic	None	MHSP
Inpatient Hospital						
Unadjusted	$672 ++*	$807 ++*	$744 ++*	$503 n+*	$329 -+*	$457
Adjusted for:						
Equitable	654 +n	727 ++	785 ++	524 n+	435 n+	474
Inequitable:						
Immutable	649 +n	736 ++	797 ++	529 n+	433 n+	496
Mutable	643 ++	722 ++	813 ++	522 n+	466 n+	497
OPD/ER Physician						
Unadjusted	41 -n	220 ++	156 ++	48 nn	41 -n	48
Adjusted for:						
Equitable	41 nn	214 ++	155 ++	46 nn	45 n+	45
Inequitable:						
Immutable	41 -n	215 ++	156 ++	47 nn	44 n+	48
Mutable	41 -n	213 ++	158 ++	46 nn	47 n+	47
Other Physician						
Unadjusted	134 n-	44 --	53 --	115 --	56 --	177
Adjusted for:						
Equitable	132 n-	41 --	55 --	117 --	61 --	179
Inequitable:						
Immutable	133 --	41 --	57 --	114 --	58 --	184
Mutable	132 --	40 --	60 --	112 --	63 --	183
Ancillaries						
Unadjusted	225 ++	212 ++	139 -+	181 ++	135 -+	132
Adjusted for:						
Equitable	220 ++	208 ++	149 n+	192 ++	146 -+	143
Inequitable:						
Immutable	214 ++	218 n+	163 -n	199 ++	144 -n	174
Mutable	211 ++	217 n+	169 -n	200 n+	152 -n	179
Total						
Unadjusted	1072	1283	1092	847	561	814
Adjusted for:						
Equitable	1047	1191	1144	879	686	841
Inequitable:						
Immutable	1037	1209	1173	889	680	901
Mutable	1026	1192	1200	879	728	906

*   The left hand column indicates the effect for proportion using the service,
     and the right hand column indicates the effect for volume of services for
     those using it.
+ = effect is greater (p<.05) than for the MHSP comparison group.
- = effect is less (p<.05) than for the MHSP comparison group.
n = no significant difference.

Chapter 10
Summary and Implications

LU ANN ADAY

RONALD M. ANDERSEN

HEALTH POLICY developments in the early part of the century led to the expansion of the U.S. health care system and to improved access for many of the traditionally medically disenfranchised segments of the U.S. population. Progress has not been without its price, however. There has been a corresponding acceleration in the rate of expenditures for medical care accompanying these changes. In the last decade public and private providers and third-party payors have responded by encouraging initiatives to cut back on the resources spent on health care and to develop innovative organizational models for the cost-effective practice of medicine. These changes may have profound impacts on the previously favorable trends of improved access for groups for whom the doors of the health care system were historically more likely to be closed, e.g., the poor, minorities, the uninsured, and/or medically "homeless."

This book provides a look at what is happening to the financing and organization of care, as experienced by consumers. Of special interest are those groups most apt to be vulnerable to restrictive medical care policies. We have, therefore, examined people's sources of medical care and insurance coverage, with special attention to traditionally disadvantaged groups, such as minorities and the poor. We have considered their needs for care, access to services, and the costs of providing these services.

The analyses summarized here provide some preliminary

answers to the questions outlined in the Health Care for the Indigent Research Agenda recently developed by the Council on Research and Development of the American Hospital Association (Council on Research and Development, AHA, 1986), and suggest the policy and health services research activities that should be developed to better inform the development of policies and programs for the indigent and other groups particularly vulnerable to shifts in U.S. health care policy.

The Approach

The analyses reported here draw upon a wide array of data representing the United States as a whole; a variety of rural, suburban, and central city communities; the poor in the one state that, at the time of the study reported here, had no federally-sponsored public insurance program for the indigent; and a city with a relatively comprehensive Medicaid program buttressed by a network of public hospitals and ambulatory care facilities. The five major data sets included in the analyses are all ones from studies supported by the Robert Wood Johnson Foundation in connection with their continuing programmatic interests in monitoring and enhancing the impact of federal and community-based organizational and financing innovations on access to medical care. These five data sets include a 1982 national telephone survey of the U.S. population; multi-site studies of eleven communities and five inner city areas in connection with evaluations of the Robert Wood Johnson-sponsored Community Hospital Program (CHP) and Municipal Health Services Program (MHSP); and surveys of the poor in the state of Arizona and New York City. Data for these studies were collected between early 1981 and late 1982, with the majority of the interviews conducted in 1982. Earlier questionnaires developed by the Center for Health Administration Studies (CHAS), the University of Chicago, formed the basis for the design of the questions asked in these studies, and, therefore, considerable comparability in the information existed across the data sets.

A framework for identifying who might be the groups *most vulnerable* to the organizational and financial changes underway in the United States guided the analysis. This framework pinpointed the relevant variables to consider in addressing who is most likely to be impacted by these changes, what are their needs, what means they potentially have available to obtain care, and what their access actually is or might be as a result of the changes underway in the U.S. health care system.

People's regular sources of medical care and insurance coverage provide the focal point for addressing these questions. Having a regular medical provider and insurance are the principal means available to patients to facilitate their care-seeking. They are also indicators of the broad organizational and financial alternatives available in the U.S. health care system for the provision and purchase of care. We also considered a set of selection variables, e.g., education, occupation, ethnicity, income, in describing who has (or selects) what types of care and coverage that correspond to the predisposing and enabling variables in Andersen's behavioral model of health services utilization (Andersen, 1968).

Need refers to indicators of who requires care the most (Andersen, 1968). A major question addressed here was whether individuals who have different means (type of insurance or regular provider) available to them for obtaining services also have different needs. A related concern was the extent to which those who had the most needs were also the most vulnerable to the proposed cutbacks in services and coverage.

The means available to particular individuals to obtain care reflect the characteristics of the health care environment in which they reside. These dimensions include both aggregate resource-availability parameters, such as physician to population ratios and per capita income of the communities in which respondents live, as well as the types of care and coverage particular individuals actually have.

Of principal concern was the extent to which actual access to care varies as a result of the types of care and coverage available to an individual. Both descriptive and multivariate analyses address the question: who has the most and least access? Access was measured by objective indicators of convenience and utilization and more subjective reports of patient satisfaction with care. Differences that were due to need were argued to be equitable or justifiable differences. The most policy-vulnerable groups are those with low access scores after adjustments for need *and* for whom the prospects of the impact of policy changes on access appear to be the least favorable.

A Summary of the Findings

The findings are summarized in the context of their implications for considering who might be most vulnerable to current and proposed changes in the organization and financing of services.

Who Has What Types of Care and Coverage?

The vast majority of Americans use private doctors as their regular source of care. These tend to be majority White individuals with better jobs and higher incomes. However, the majority of traditionally disadvantaged groups, such as minority and poor individuals, *also* use private doctors as their regular sources of care. While private doctors are the *modal* group for most segments of the population, they are *less likely* to be the principal source of care for the disadvantaged. The CHP groups were generally utilized by patients whose profile looked very similar to those using private doctors' offices. Thus, while the CHPs attracted some poor, minority, and uninsured persons, the groups they served could not be characterized as a particularly policy-vulnerable population.

For low-income people, especially those who reside in inner city areas, hospital outpatient departments (OPDs) are also important sources of routine medical care. This is rooted in the tradition of large teaching and research hospitals providing free or low-cost care to the indigent to ensure a caseload of patients for ongoing medical education and research efforts at those institutions. The importance of OPDs for the poor is mirrored in the national study findings, and reinforced by the results for the sample of the low-income population in Arizona and the urban inner city universes represented in the New York City and MHSP studies. Multivariate analyses of the people who use OPDs regularly bear out that they are apt to have poorer health; be Black, unemployed, inner city residents; have lived in their community shorter periods of time; and have public coverage only or no insurance at all.

Though the percentage of those who use hospital emergency rooms (ERs) regularly for care is quite small overall nationally (2 percent), this represents almost five million Americans who can name no place they regularly go for medical care other than a nearby hospital's ER. People who frequent the ER are on average younger than those using OPDs, although few children are regular users of ERs. The importance of this source for inner city residents was illustrated in the MHSP sample, which had the largest percentage (5 percent) using ERs regularly relative to any of the other samples.

The extensive use of neighborhood health centers and other government clinics by the indigent is reflected in the particularly high proportion of the low-income Arizona sample (15 percent) who reported these as their regular source of medical care. Multivariate analyses confirmed that people with lower socioeconomic statuses are more likely to use these sources. The MHSP, representing a special type of publicly sponsored primary health center, also served the most economically disadvantaged groups in their communities.

Indigent patients who have traditionally used hospital OPDs or ERs or publicly subsidized clinics may be particularly vulnerable as financial constraints on these sources of care increase. Reasons for the growing financial problems of these institutions include reductions in federal support for community health centers and manpower redistribution programs; increased transfers of unfunded patients to public teaching hospitals; reduced federal support for public-pay patients; and a heightened interest on the part of private hospitals in maximizing collectible accounts and minimizing their burden of uncompensated care.

One out of ten (some twenty-four million) Americans do not have a regular place they go to for medical care. People who report having no regular source of care at all are more likely to be older, male, in better health overall, relative newcomers to their community, and especially to be uninsured. Most of these individuals say they would go to a doctor's office should they need care. Still, a third to a half of the respondents in the several studies could not name any place they would go to, should the need arise. Two-thirds or more of the reasons given for not having a regular medical provider appeared to be voluntary — they did not feel they needed one; were seldom sick; or got care regularly, but did not identify one particular place as their primary provider. However, around a third of the reasons cited suggest that not having a regular provider was not a voluntary decision. A reason cited most frequently in the low-income Arizona sample was that the person "can't afford a regular source." Other seemingly involuntary responses included that they had recently moved, their old doctor was no longer available, and/or that "they did not know any doctor."

Some "medically homeless" appear more vulnerable than others. Those who have no place they know of they could go for care should the need arise and/or are involuntarily without a source, because of financial or other access barriers, would appear to be *most* vulnerable to efforts to restrict services in a given community or delivery setting. Others without a routine point of entry, but who do not consider themselves in need of regular care and/or have an idea of where to go if necessary, should be viewed as less vulnerable from a policy point of view.

Insurance is another principal determinant of who is likely to have the best access to medical care. The vast majority of Americans have some type of private insurance coverage. Public insurance (especially Medicaid) is a more important form of coverage for the low–income and inner city populations. Many elderly have private coverage supplementary to Medicare.

The multivariate analyses point out the sharp contrast in the characteristics of those people under sixty-five years of age who have public coverage only compared to those who have private insurance. The publicly insured are more likely to have poor health, be minority, have less than a high school education, be poor, unemployed or working in low-status occupations, and use hospital OPDs regularly or have no regular place to go for routine medical care. Similarly, the elderly who have Medicare only are more likely than those who have some type of private supplementary coverage to be minority, poor and have no regular source of medical care.

Cutbacks in the Medicaid program have already reduced the proportion of the poor who are insured. Changes in the Medicare program portend greater cost-sharing on the part of beneficiaries. Analyses of those individuals who are solely dependent on public insurance programs indicate they are likely to have greater needs and fewer personal resources to assume a larger share of the burden of their health care costs than those with some sort of private insurance.

From 11 to 14 percent of the samples, with the exception of Arizona, reported being uninsured. In the Arizona low-income sample, where no Medicaid program existed, approximately one-third reported having no insurance at all. A disproportionate number of the uninsured in all the studies were, in fact, low-income. Multivariate analyses of the uninsured bear out that they have poorer perceived health. They are more likely to be unemployed or work in low-status jobs, be poor, live in central cities, and use hospital OPDs or ERs regularly or report having no place they go to for routine medical care. Of the innovative primary care programs we examined in this study, CHP clinics, on average, served about the same proportion of uninsured as were found in the community as a whole. MHSP clinics, however, included relatively larger proportions of the uninsured among their regular users.

Evidence shows that the number of uninsured has grown. As mentioned earlier, with the accompanying stricter eligibility requirements for the Medicaid program in many states, and recessions and resultant layoffs in many American communities over the last few years, larger numbers of the poor and non-poor have become ineligible for either public or private coverage. Those without any type of insurance appear to be a particularly vulnerable group in the context of increasing financial and institutional constraints in the U.S. health care system.

When we look at combinations of care and coverage, we find that people with a private doctor *and* some private health insurance are more likely to have higher incomes and educational levels and less likely to be minority than those without any insurance coverage or a regular source of care. Those with no identifiable source of either care or coverage represent a relatively small proportion of the total U.S. population (2 percent), but might be expected to be the most vulnerable to current health policy developments in the organization and financing of care.

Who Are the Medically Needy?

Descriptive analyses of a variety of measures of need indicate that samples of hospital OPD users had higher proportions reporting fair or poor health, more frequent health worries, more disability days, and mean numbers of symptoms, compared particularly to people who had private physicians or no regular source of care. These differences were borne out in all five studies. Independent physician ratings of the severity of symptoms reported in the CHP and MHSP studies similarly confirmed that the symptoms reported by OPD users were more serious than those reported by people who went to private physicians, and that those experienced by people who did not have a regular source of care at all were much less serious as well. Despite the sense of urgency in the ER, its regular users are, according to most measures we examined, in better health than the regular OPD patients. These data establish then that the neediest or most medically vulnerable group is probably patients who use hospital OPDs.

Many of those who do not have a regular source of care report themselves to be in good health and not "in need" of a regular source of medical care. However, those who are involuntarily without a regular source have poorer health and appear, therefore, to be a more medically vulnerable group. Regular users of both the CHPs and MHSPs generally appeared to be in as good or better health than people with other sources of care, but in poorer health than those reporting *no* regular source of care.

People under sixty-five with public coverage alone or some combination of public and private coverage are most likely to report having fair or poor health, more worry and disability, more symptoms and more severe symptoms than those with private coverage alone or no insurance at all. Among the uninsured, however, the poor are much more likely to report poorer perceived health and more disability than the non-poor. For those sixty-five and over, people with combinations of public and private coverage are in better health than those with public coverage alone. It seems, then, that the elderly who can afford supplementary coverage to Medicare are also in better health.

Persons with public insurance *and* a hospital OPD as a regular source of care had the poorest health overall. These people, as well as those in poor health who are involuntarily without a regular point of entry to the health care system, or who are poor *and* uninsured would seem to be particularly vulnerable groups, should their access to needed care be reduced.

The examination of the actual access patterns for these and other groups controlling for need will illuminate the extent to which they might be particularly vulnerable to further constraints in the organization and financing of medical care in the United States.

Who Has the Most and Least Access and Why?

A variety of indicators of the convenience, utilization of, and satisfaction with services were examined to determine the actual access profiles of individuals with different types of care and coverage.

An analysis of mean office waiting times confirmed that regular users of hospital OPDs and ERs tended to average much longer waits than those who went to see private physicians. People who had public coverage only, many of whom use hospital OPD and ER facilities, averaged longer waiting times than those with some type of private insurance. Waiting times were also longer for minority and poor patients. The convenience of care then continues to be less for these traditionally and potentially policy vulnerable groups.

The proportion having actually seen a doctor in the year was much lower for people who did not have a regular source of medical care or insurance coverage. The multivariate analyses confirm that need is an important predictor of whether or not care is sought. However, the mutable policy-relevant correlates of care and coverage remain as important determinants of whether or not a provider is apt to be seen, regardless of need. The analyses of the special samples demonstrated the portion of poor people seeing a physician within a year in NYC (with a comprehensive Medicaid program) was considerably higher than in Arizona (before any Medicaid program was in place). Further, our examination of a range of Hispanic and Black populations across the country points out wide discrepancies in access to physicians. It highlights that while minority groups may generally have access problems, their vulnerability varies a great deal, depending on where they live and the characteristics of the health care systems in their communities.

Once a physician is contacted, it is apparent that need is a particularly important predictor of a patient's overall number of visits. People under sixty-five with public coverage only appear to average more visits than those with private insurance, however, after controlling for need. These higher utilization rates for the publicly insured may reflect doctor shopping, discontinuous or poorly coordinated follow-up care or the use of the medical care system for psychosocially–related problems emanating from the stresses of their lower socioeconomic standing — situations which current efforts to enroll the poor in more comprehensive, managed systems of care are purportedly attempting to address. In fact, while the NYC poor (apparently in a more comprehensive system) were more likely to see a doctor than the Arizona poor, they had *fewer* visits once they sought care than did the indigent in the state of Arizona.

As with physician contacts, the rates of hospitalization are much lower for people who do not have a regular source of medical care or coverage individual. Need is certainly a primary determinant of whether or not an individual is hospitalized. Even controlling for need, however, these care and coverage factors continue to have a significant impact on the decision to admit a patient. Blacks are less likely to be admitted than Whites, given comparable need and other characteristics. Once admitted, need continues to be a primary determinant of the patient's length of stay. Still, the multivariate analyses demonstrated that people who do not have insurance are much more likely to be discharged sooner, even after taking need into account.

The role of the social and enabling factors in influencing decisions about whom to hospitalize and how long they stay need to be monitored carefully in a rationing-oriented health care environment. For example, people who regularly use OPDs tend to have relatively longer lengths of stay and a relatively larger proportion of their total services consumed on a hospital inpatient, rather than outpatient, basis. OPD users, particularly those who are publicly insured, as well as the uninsured, contribute significantly to many hospitals' uncompensated care problems. Hence, they become prime candidates for "dumping" as fiscal constraints on these institutions increase.

The evidence from the analysis of the special samples points to the relatively low inpatient hospital use of regular users of the more comprehensive, managed systems of care. For example, the NYC poor are less likely to be hospitalized than the low–income people in the United States as a whole, and the MHSP and CHP patients are generally admitted less often than persons who use other regular sources of care in their communities. This may reduce their vulnerability to policy efforts to constrain inpatient use, since they are already less dependent on inpatient services.

Rates of use relative to need and selected preventive procedures remain less for those who do not have a regular source of care or health insurance. One's health status is an important predictor of whether or not they have had a blood pressure reading taken in the year. People who are better-educated and have higher incomes are more likely to have had their blood pressure checked. Even controlling for these and other factors, people who have a private physician are much more likely to have had this procedure in the past year. Less likely to have blood pressure checks are those who use ERs or some other type of clinic regularly, or do not have any place they usually go for care. Similarly, people who do not have any type of public or private insurance coverage are less likely to have had their blood pressure checked than those with private insurance. The importance of education, as well as having a regular source of care and/or private insurance coverage, in predicting whether women will have had a pap smear or breast exam in the year, is borne out in the multivariate analyses as well. Enrolling people in more health maintenance-oriented care arrangements may then enhance their access to these important preventive procedures.

People are more dissatisfied with costs than any other aspect of their care. It appears that people with public insurance or who use hospital OPDs or ERs regularly have the lowest direct out-of-pocket outlays. These individuals may become increasingly vulnerable to decision-making about who the institution can afford to treat as the financial constraints on hospitals increase. Dissatisfaction with care overall in the most recent encounter with a physician is associated with being younger, in poorer health, a male, new to the community, using hospital OPDs or ERs as one's regular source of care, or having no regular care source. Regular users of CHP and MHSP clinics appear more satisfied with their care than other patients in the community, except those who use private doctors. CHP patients do not differ significantly from patients of private doctors while MHSP patients appear somewhat less satisfied.

What Are the Costs of Different Sources of Regular Care?

The expenditure analyses from the MHSP study emphasize that regular uses of hospital OPDs and ERs have the highest total expenditures, even when adjustments are made for their needs and other inequitable characteristics. The expenses for these patients are high because of relatively large inpatient outlays and the receipt of ambulatory care in expensive hospital outpatient settings. OPD and ER patients, therefore, appear particularly vulnerable to cost containment policies. They are not only more likely to be poor and dependent on the public sector for financing. They also receive costly care from the hospital sector, which is most likely to be the target of policies to contain medical care costs.

People without a regular source of care have the lowest medical care expenses even after taking into account their relatively good health. Their vulnerability to future restrictive policies rests largely on their lack of health insurance to finance needed care. As competitive pressures and reduced public funding proceed to limit unfunded or partially funded care, access to services for those without a regular source may be especially affected.

People who use private doctors' offices have total per capita expenses in between the hospital users and those without a regular source of care. They are probably least policy vulnerable since they on average have the largest incomes, the most comprehensive insurance, and moderate medical expenses. However, it should be remembered that private doctors are the modal source of care for most subgroups in the population, including the poor, the publicly insured and uninsured, and minority persons. Thus, policies to limit payments to private doctors for groups such as these can increase the vulnerability of large numbers of regular users of private physicians' services.

The regular users of MHSP and other public clinics have the lowest average medical expenses, except for people without a regular source. These innovative forms of organizing care are themselves vulnerable, in the sense that they often receive public or private subsidies that are subject to cuts during periods of budgetary constraint. However, their relatively good track record in de-emphasizing expensive hospital services and containing overall medical costs may make them appear relatively attractive to public and private funders in a period of limited resources.

In sum, who appears to be most vulnerable to current changes underway in the U.S. health care system? People who use hospital OPDs as their regular source of care, especially those who only have some form of public insurance coverage or no insurance, are prime candidates for dumping or underservice in the increasingly constrained health care environment. Americans who do not have a regular source of medical care, particularly those in poor health who want one but can't afford it, should be of particular concern in emerging initiatives to develop managed systems of care for the indigent. The uninsured are least able to afford the high cost of medical care. The uninsured poor particularly tend to have the poorest health. It is these individuals who should receive special attention in efforts to cover the medically indigent who slip through the cracks of existing public and private systems of coverage.

Implications for Policy and Further Research

In this final section we will briefly review what we believe to be the key policy implications of this study. In addition, we will note some instances where additional research might better focus policies to improve care and coverage for the U.S. population as a whole, as well as for particularly medically disadvantaged subgroups.

— Some of the alternative ways of managing care, as exemplified by the Community Hospital and Municipal Health Services Programs, are providing promising avenues to maximize access and contain costs. They (especially MHSP) also demonstrate the capacity to serve the disadvantaged. We need to specify what elements of these alternative programs impact most directly on access and costs. It is also crucial to understand how alternative, as well as traditional, sources of care ultimately affect quality and health status outcomes as well.

— Since private doctors' offices and clinics continue to be the regular source of care used by most Americans, attention should be given to what aspects consumers find most appealing. For example, patients are attracted by the personal nature of care in the doctor's office. Overhead costs tend to be lower in these settings as well, particularly compared to large-scale (especially hospital outpatient) settings. Research could help inform us as to whether and how a personalized doctor-patient relationship can be attained in increasingly large and bureaucratized ambulatory care settings, such as HMOs. We should also further examine the cost and quality tradeoffs between providing front-line medical care in more primary care-oriented versus more technology-intensive delivery systems.

—Some mechanism needs to be found to provide health insurance to the uninsured, since the majority of them cannot realistically afford health insurance and their need for health care is great, relative to their use of services. Additional studies need to be done of the probable and actual *costs* to insure this population, and on the most cost-effective *means* to provide them government or private insurance-based third party benefits.

—Additional means for supplementing Medicare coverage would be helpful, since it is clear that the elderly most in need of supplementary coverage (the low–income elderly) are least likely to have it. Now, they spend their own limited resources to supplement Medicare and become Medicaid recipients, once their resources are exhausted. We need to know more about the personal and societal costs of this spend-down process.

—Since the majority of people without a regular source of care do not feel the need of one and are in relatively good health, policy should be directed toward the "medically homeless" in poor health and/or actively wanting to obtain care. More information is needed as to how and why people do or do not select a regular source of care and what mechanisms can be encouraged to better link individuals without a regular source to a "preferred" *and* appropriate provider.

—OPDs and ERs should be de-emphasized as regular sources of primary care. They are expensive, inconvenient, and more likely to elicit unfavorable ratings from their patients than other sources of care. However, more careful evaluation would help to sort out the functions that these institutions best serve. For example, OPDs serve sick and disadvantaged persons. Can, and will, other sources of care do a better job of caring for these people? Can those now served by OPDs in teaching hospitals in inner cities obtain care of comparable quality from other sources in their neighborhoods? ERs serve a less sick, higher income, more mobile population. Can other organizations (such as "emergicenters" or "urgicenters") meet the needs of these people as well? If ERs lose their primary care business, will it adversely affect the quality, price, or availability of their "real emergency" services?

—The diversity of needs and medical care use patterns of minorities in different communities points out the need for health policy to be flexible and responsive to local markets. The challenge for health policy is to encourage innovations that may respond more efficiently and effectively to local needs.

Current changes underway in the organization and financing of care in the United States are apt to have profound impacts on potential and realized access to medical care. The analyses reported here help identify the groups that are most likely to be vulnerable to these transformations in care and coverage, and the resultant implications for their access to the U.S. health care system.

Appendix A
Description of Variables

CHRISTOPHER S. LYTTLE

IT IS NOT POSSIBLE to reprint all of the survey questionnaires in this appendix. However, except for the New York City Access Survey, each of them is available in some published source. The 1982 National Access Survey questionnaire is included as Appendix F in Aday, et al. (1984); the questionnaire for the Arizona study is Appendix D in Harris (1983) which is the data collection agency's report to The Robert Wood Johnson Foundation; the questionnaire for the Community Hospital Program (CHP) Access Evaluation is Appendix D in Aday, et al. (1985); and the Municipal Health Services Program (MHSP) Access Evaluation questionnaire is Appendix C in Fleming and Andersen (1986).

This appendix provides the reader with the text of the original questions for the 1982 National Access Survey, and it gives some indication of whether the item is available in the other studies in a largely identical (no parentheses around question number) or slightly modified form (question number enclosed in parentheses). When appropriate, categories of constructed variables are provided as well. Items may be located in any number of sections of the questionnaires. Item numbers with no alphabetic prefix are located in the main body of the respondent questionnaire; items listed as "LF" or "LF" and a number, come from the family "Listing Form"; items with an "F" prefix are located in the family "Factuals" which are asked only once for each family; and items starting with an "S" are part of the screener section of the questionnaire for determining eligibility for inclusion in the survey.

NATIONAL	ARIZONA	CHP	MHSP	NYC

I.   *SELECTION VARIABLES*

   A.   PREDISPOSING

A.1.   Age (continuous)

Item:	LF	LF	LF	LF	LF

A.2.   Age (categorical, derived from continuous age)

Values: (0) less than 1 year
             (1) 1–5 years
             (2) 6–17 years
             (3) 18–34 years
             (4) 35–54 years
             (5) 55–64 years
             (6) 65 or more years

A.3.   Sex

Item:	LF	LF	LF	LF	LF

A.4.   Education of Adult Respondent

Item:	F3a	F3a	(72)	(84)	F2a

What was the last grade of school that you (s/he) completed?

a. No formal schooling
b. First through 7th grade
c. 8th grade
d. Some high school
f. High school graduate
g. Some college
h. Two-year college graduate
i. Four-year college graduate
j. Postgraduate

   Trade/technical/vocational after high school (ask for details, and code into one of the above categories).

NATIONAL	ARIZONA	CHP	MHSP	NYC

A.5. Employment Status of Adult Respondent

Item: F3b   F3b   (73)   (88)   F2b

Which of the following best describes your (her/his) current employment situation? (READ LIST)

a. Working full-time
b. Working part-time
c. Laid off or on strike
d. Unemployed but looking for work
e. Unemployed and not looking for work
f. Retired
g. Unable to work — disabled
h. Keeping house
i. Full-time student

A.6. Occupation of Adult Respondent

Item: F3c   F3c   (76a)   (90)   F2c

What type of work do you (does s/he) do?

a. Professional
b. Manager, official
c. Proprietor (small business)
d. Clerical worker
e. Sales worker
f. Skilled craftsman, foreman
g. Operative, unskilled laborer (except farm)
h. Service worker
i. Farmer, farm manager, farm laborer
j. Military service
k. Other (SPECIFY)

NATIONAL	ARIZONA	CHP	MHSP	NYC

A.7. Education of Main Wage Earner

Item:	F2a	F2a	(65)	(84)	F1b

What was the last grade of school that the main wage earner completed?

Same categories as A.4.

A.8. Employment Status of Main Wage Earner

Item:	F2b	F2b	(66)	(88)	F1c

Which of the following best describes (her/his) current employment situation: Is (s/he) READ LIST)?

Same categories as A.5.

A.9. Occupation of Main Wage Earner

Item:	F2c	F2c	(69a)	(90)	F1d

What type of work does (s/he) do?

Same categories as A.6.

A.10. Minority Status

Item:	F8	(F8)	(63)	(76)	F8

Do you (does s/he) consider yourself (himself/herself) — white, black, oriental, or what?

a. White
b. Black
c. Oriental/Asian or Pacific Islander
d. American Indian or Alaskan native

A.11. Hispanic Origin

Item:	F9	F9	(64)	(77)	F9

NATIONAL	ARIZONA	CHP	MHSP	NYC

Are you (is s/he) of Hispanic origin, or not?

A.12. Race — Reduced Form

Values: (1) White, Non-Minority
(2) Black
(3) Hispanic
(4) Other
(9) Missing

A.13. Family Size

Item:	LF count	S1b	LF 6	LF G	S1a

B.   ENABLING

B.1.   Family Income (continuous)

Item:	—	—	70	(96,98)	—

Now we need to know how much your family's total
combined income from all family members was during
the past twelve months — that is, yours and (REFER TO
LISTING FORM AND READ NAMES OF ALL
FAMILY MEMBERS). This includes income from all
sources, such as wages, salaries, social security or
retirement benefits, interest or dividends, rent from
property and so forth.

B.2.   Family Income (categorical)

Item:	F6b1-9	F6b1-18	(70A)	(96A,98A)	S1b

Which of the following income categories best describe
your total 1981 family income? Please be sure to include

NATIONAL	ARIZONA	CHP	MHSP	NYC

income from welfare, Social Security, pensions and investments, as well as any wages and salary or income from your own business.

Note:

Category list is different for each family size in the National and Arizona studies, with category boundaries allowing identification of poverty level or Arizona Health Care Cost Containment System (AHCCCS) eligibility level, respectively.

B.3.   Family Income – Reduced Form (High, Medium, Low)

Values: (1) LE $7,200
             (2) $7,201–25,000 ($12,600 in Arizona)
             (3) GT $25,000   ($12,600 in Arizona)

B.4.   Poverty Level

Values: (1) LT 1
             (2) 1.0–1.5
             (3) GT 1.5

Note:

These cutoffs are relative to the 1981 national poverty level, except in Arizona where cutoffs are relative to the AHCCCS eligibility levels. Poverty level cutoffs are not available for the New York City survey.

II.   *NEED VARIABLES*

A.1.   Self-perceived health

Item:	2	1	28	53	2

Would you say that your (her/his) health, in general, is excellent, good, fair, or poor?

	NATIONAL	ARIZONA	CHP	MHSP	NYC

A.2. Worry

Item: —   —   29   54   —

Over the past year has your health caused you a great deal of worry, some worry, hardly any worry, or no worry at all?

A.3. Bed days in last year

Item: 3a   2a   (47)   (55)   3a

How many days *altogether* during the past year, that is, since (DATE ONE YEAR AGO) 1981, did you (s/he) stay in bed more than half of the day because of illness or injury? Include any days you (s/he) stayed in the hospital.

A.4. Non-hospital days in bed during last year

Bed days (II.A.3.) minus hospital bed days (V.B.19.).

A.5. Other disability days in last year

Item: 3b   2b   (48)   56   3b

Not counting the days in bed, how many days during the past year, that is since (DATE ONE YEAR AGO) 1981, did you (s/he) have to cut down on the things you usually do (s/he usually does) for more than half of the day because of illness or injury?

A.6. Total disability days in last year

Sum of non-hospital bed days and other disability days.

A.7. Symptoms

Item: —   —   30   58   —

NATIONAL   ARIZONA   CHP   MHSP   NYC

Please look at the symptoms on Card D and we'll go over them together. These questions refer to your experiences during the past twelve months, since (DATE ONE YEAR AGO). (FOR EACH SYMPTOM, ASK:) Did you experience (SYMPTOM) at any time this year?

A Cough any time during the day or night which lasted for three weeks?

B Sudden feelings of weakness or faintness?

C Feeling tired for weeks at a time for no special reason?

D Frequent headaches?

E Diarrhea (loose bowel movements) for four or five days?

F Shortness of breath even after light work?

G Waking up with stiff or aching joints or muscles?

H Pain or swelling in any joints during the day?

I Frequent backaches?

J If 6+ YEARS OF AGE: Unexplained loss of over ten pounds in weight?

K Repeated pains in or near the heart?

L Repeated indigestion or upset stomach?

M Sore throat or runny nose with a fever as high as 100° F. for at least two days?

N Abdominal pains (pains in the belly or gut) for at least a couple of days?

O Any infections, irritations, or pains in the eyes or ears?

A.8. Number of symptoms

This is a simple count of the number of symptoms reported.

A.9. Symptom Severity Index

NATIONAL	ARIZONA	CHP	MHSP	NYC

The Symptom Severity Index reflects the ratings of a panel of physicians of the proportion of people with a symptom who should see a physician for it. The ratings were summed across all symptoms reported to obtain the summary index. See Appendix E in Aday, et al. (1980) for a discussion of how the physician ratings were obtained.

III.   *SYSTEM VARIABLES*

A.   RESIDENCE

A.1.   Location (FIPS Code)

All studies except CHP and MHSP identified responses as originating from a Federal Information Processing Standard (FIPS) unit. Generally this is a county, but sometimes it is a city, and in the case of New York City boroughs are identified. CHP and MHSP identified responses by "site," which were service areas for particular facilities being evaluated. All MHSP and most CHP sites lie completely within a FIPS unit. Those CHP sites not completely within a FIPS unit were linked to the unit which represented most of the service area.

A.2.   Location – Reduced Form (Region)

Values: (1) Northeast
        (2) North Central
        (3) South
        (4) West

A.3.   Residence (Central City, SMSA, etc.)

Item:	FIPS	FIPS	Site	—	—

	NATIONAL	ARIZONA	CHP	MHSP	NYC

Note:

MHSP and NYC are considered Central City by definition. CHP is coded by site with farm/non-farm distinction in non-SMSA areas based on question LF10.

A.4.   Residence — Reduced Form

Values: (1) Central City
(2) SMSA, Other
(3) Non-SMSA, Non-farm
(4) Non-SMSA, Farm

A.5.   Length of residence in the city, neighborhood, community

Item:	F7a	F7a	(71)	(78)	(F6a)

For how many years have you lived in this community?

(1) Less than 2 years
(2) 2 to 5 years
(3) 6 to 10 years
(4) 11 to 15 years
(5) 16 to 20 years
(6) More than 20 years

B.   AREA RESOURCE FILE (ARF)
(U.S. Department of Commerce, 1984)

B.1.   Physician Supply

Total 1981 non-federal, patient care physicians per 1000 1980 census population.

B.2.   Per capita income

1980 per capita income.

NATIONAL	ARIZONA	CHP	MHSP	NYC

IV. *MEANS VARIABLES*

A. REGULAR SOURCE

A.1. Is there a regular source of care?

Item:	5a	4a	1	1	5a

Is there one person or place in particular you (s/he) usually go(es) to when you are (s/he is) sick or (s/he) want(s) advice about your (her/his) health?

A.2. Description of regular source of care

Item:	6a	(5a)	(7)	(2)	6a

Where do you (does s/he) usually go — to a doctor's office, a clinic, a hospital or some other place?

IF CLINIC: Is it a private clinic; a hospital outpatient clinic; a company or union clinic; a school clinic, a neighborhood or government-sponsored clinic; or any other clinic not connected with a hospital?

IF HOSPITAL: Is it a hospital outpatient clinic or a hospital emergency room?

IF SOME OTHER PLACE: What type of place is it?

A.3. Is it an HMO?

Item:	6b	(5b)	—	—	6b

Is that place a health maintenance organization or HMO; that is, a place you go to for all or most medical care, which is paid for by a fixed monthly or annual amount?

NATIONAL	ARIZONA	CHP	MHSP	NYC

A.4. Regular Source of Care — Reduced Form

Values: (1) Private Doctor's Office or Clinic
(2) Hospital OPD
(3) Hospital ER
(4) Other
(5) No Regular Care
(6) No Information

A.5. If no "regular place", is there a "might go" place?

Item:	5c	(4d)	(3)	—	5c

Is there a medical doctor or osteopath you (s/he) *might* go to if you (s/he) needed medical care?

A.6. Description of place "might go"

Item:	6a	(4f)	(4)	—	6a

Same text as A.2.

A.7. Is it an HMO?

Item:	6b	(5b)	—	—	6b

Same text as A.3.

B.   INSURANCE COVERAGE

B.1. Any insurance coverage?

Item:	—	—	59	—	—

Are you covered by any of the health plans listed on Card 1?

NATIONAL	ARIZONA	CHP	MHSP	NYC

Note:

Presence of insurance was derived from B.2.–B.14. for those studies not asking directly.

B.2.–B.14.   Type of insurance coverage.

Now I'd like to talk about the different kinds of health plans or health insurance that people have, including those provided by the government. As I read each of the following health plans, please tell me whether you are (s/he is) covered by it.

B.2.   County paid medical care?

Item:	—	27	—	—	—

B.3.   Health insurance through work or union?

Item:	22	27	60	(11)	27

B.4.   Health insurance through some other group?

Item:	22	27	(60)	(11)	27

B.5.   Health insurance bought directly by yourself (himself/herself) or your (his/her) family?

Item:	22	27	60	(12)	27

B.6.   Medicare A, that pays hospital bills for people aged 65 and over and for some disabled people?

Item:	22	27	(60)	9a	27

B.7.   Medicare B, that pays doctor's bills for people aged 65 and over and for some disabled people?

Item:	22	27	(60)	(9c)	27

	NATIONAL	ARIZONA	CHP	MHSP	NYC

B.8. Medicaid or Public Aid?

Item:	22	—	60	(10)	27

B.9. Prepaid group practice or HMO (that is, a place you go for all or most medical care which is paid for by a fixed monthly or annual amount)?

Item:	22	27	(60)	(13)	(27)

B.10. Another clinic or health care center where you (s/he) can get care at no cost or at reduced rates?

Item:	22	27	60	(13)	27

B.11. Any other place? (SPECIFY)

Item:	22	27	60	(13)	27

B.12. Veteran's Administration?

Item:	—	—	60	(13)	—

B.13. Coverage for military personnel and their dependents (CHAMPUS)?

Item:	—	—	60	(13)	—

B.14. School Insurance?

Item:	—	—	60	(13)	—

B.15. Insurance Coverage — Reduced Form

Values: (1) Public Only (Medicare, Medicaid, County)
        (2) Private Only (All other except B.10.)
        (3) Public and Private
        (4) None
        (9) Missing

NATIONAL	ARIZONA	CHP	MHSP	NYC

V.   *ACTUAL ACCESS VARIABLES*

A.   CONVENIENCE

A.1.   Waiting Time

Item: 7f   (13f)   (23)   73   7g

How long did you have to wait to see the doctor once you (s/he) got there?

B.   UTILIZATION – Contact and Volume

B.1.   M.D. Contact in last year (Y/N)

Item: 7a,8   13a,14   (52)   (30)   7a,8

What was the month and year of your (her/his) most recent medical visit – when you (s/he) actually saw a doctor in an office or at a clinic?

Did you (s/he) *see* or *talk* to a doctor any time during the past twelve months, that is since (DATE ONE YEAR AGO) 1981? This includes visits to the doctor and any visit to a nurse or other medical person on the doctor's staff, instead of the doctor.

B.2.-B.15.   Visits in last year

How many of each of the following kinds of visits did you (s/he) have with a doctor or doctor's assistant during the past twelve months, that is, since (DATE ONE YEAR AGO) 1981?

B.2.   House calls by a doctor of doctor's assistant

Item: 10   (16)   (53e)   —   10

B.3.   Visits to a doctor's office or private clinic

Item: 10   16   53a   (37)   10

	NATIONAL	ARIZONA	CHP	MHSP	NYC
B.4. Visits to a group practice					
Item:	—	—	53b	—	—
B.5. Visits to a county clinic					
Item:	—	16	—	—	—
B.6. Visits to a non-county clinic					
Item:	—	16	—	—	—
B.7. Visits to a company or union clinic					
Item:	10	16	—	—	10
B.8. Visits to a school clinic					
Item:	10	—	—	—	10
B.9. Visits to a neighborhood or government-sponsored clinic					
Item:	10	—	—	(37)	10
B.10. Visits to a hospital outpatient clinic					
Item:	10	—	53	(37)	10
B.11. Visits as a hospital inpatient					
Item:	—	—	—	37	—
B.12. Visits to a hospital emergency room					
Item:	10	—	53	(37)	10
B.13. Visits to a county emergency room					
Item:	—	16	—	—	—

NATIONAL	ARIZONA	CHP	MHSP	NYC

B.14. Other (non-county) emergency room visits

Item: —   16   —   —   —

B.15. Visits to any other place for medical care, other than when you may have been a patient overnight in a hospital (SPECIFY)

Item: 10   16   (53)   (37)   10

B.16. Sum of Physician Visits

Summation of items B.2. through B.15.

B.17. Hospitalizations in last year (Y/N)

Item: 17a   22a   (49)   (18)   18a

Have you (has s/he) been a patient overnight in a hospital during the past twelve months, since (DATE ONE YEAR AGO) 1981?

B.18. Numbers of admissions

Item: 17b   22b   (50)   (sum(19))   18b

How many times were you (was s/he) admitted to a hospital since (DATE ONE YEAR AGO) 1981?

B.19. Number of nights

Item: 17c   22c   (51)   (sum(22))   18c

Altogether, how many nights did you (s/he) stay in a hospital during that period, that is since (DATE ONE YEAR AGO) 1981?

NATIONAL	ARIZONA	CHP	MHSP	NYC

B.20. Visit mix (inpatient vs. outpatient)

To construct standardized units for looking at the rate of hospital use to total use, all hospital days were multiplied by 5.3. This multiplier reflects the relative value of inpatient to outpatient visits, and is derived from American Hospital Association data (AHA, 1980). These adjusted units of use were then added to total outpatient visits to yield a total use figure. The rate of inpatient to total use reflects the rate of mean adjusted hospital days to the mean adjusted total use (adjusted hospital days plus the outpatient use units).

B.21. Visit mix (ER-OPD vs. other)

This estimate reflects the ratio of the mean number of visits to a hospital outpatient department or emergency room to the mean total number of visits (excluding phone calls and hospital inpatient contacts) for those who had at least one visit to the doctor in the year.

C. SATISFACTION

During the last visit for medical care, were you completely satisfied, somewhat satisfied, or not at all satisfied with (READ EACH ITEM)?

C.1. The amount of time you had to wait to see the doctor, once there

Item:	7gb	(13hb)	(27c)	75c	7ab

C.2. The out-of-pocket cost for the medical care received, that is, the cost not paid by insurance

Item:	7ge	13he	(27e)	(75e)	7ae

C.3. This visit to the doctor, overall

Item:	7gg	(13hg)	(27h)	75h	7ag

NATIONAL	ARIZONA	CHP	MHSP	NYC

D. TYPE OF SERVICE

D.1. Preventative measures (within year)

In the past twelve months, that is, since (DATE ONE YEAR AGO) 1981, have you (READ EACH ITEM), or not?

Had a blood pressure reading

Item:	4a	3a	56b	—	4a

WOMEN ONLY: Had a pap smear test for cancer

Item:	4c	3c	56e	—	4c

WOMEN ONLY: Had a breast examination by a doctor

Item:	4d	3d	56f	—	4d

D.2. Use-Disability Ratio

The use-disability ratio (physician visits per 100 days of disability) is computed by dividing the mean number of physician visits for those who have between one and 100 (inclusive) disability days in the year by their mean disability days, and then multiplying the result by 100. See V.B.16. "Sum of Physician Visits" for a definition of the contacts included in the numerator of the ratio; and II.A.6. "Total disability days in last year" for a definition of the days constituting the denominator. The ratio is limited to persons who report no more than 100 disability days to ensure that mostly short-term, acute illness episodes are considered in the analyses. See Aday, et al. (1980) for a fuller description of the ratio.

E. EXPENDITURES

Expenditure data were available in detail for only the MHSP survey. The information provided directly by the respondents was extensively verified and supplemented using external

NATIONAL	ARIZONA	CHP	MHSP	NYC

sources. For a full description of this process see Chapter 9 in this volume and Chapter 7 in Fleming and Andersen (1986).

E.1. Hospital inpatient

Item:	—	—	—	26	—

How much was the total hospital bill? (IF "DK", ASK:) Can you estimate the approximate amount?

E.2. Ambulatory OPD and ER

Item:	—	—	—	37A	—

How much was the total bill for all of these visits to (DOCTOR)? (IF "DK", ASK:) Can you estimate the approximate amount?

E.3. Other ambulatory physician

Item:	—	—	—	37A	—

Same question as E.2.

E.4. All other

Item:	—	—	—	47,48	—

Are any of the costs for (SERVICE) paid for by insurance or government programs?

(Not including what insurance pays) How much did or will (you/PERSON) have to pay for (SERVICE)? (If "DK", ASK:) Can you estimate the approximate amount?

References

Aday, Lu Ann, et al. *Health Care in the U.S.: Equitable for Whom?* Beverly Hills: Sage Publications. 1980.

Aday, Lu Ann, et al. *Access to Medical Care in the U.S.: Who Has it, Who Doesn't.* Chicago: Pluribus Press, Inc. 1984.

Aday, Lu Ann, et al. *Hospital-Physician Sponsored Primary Care: Marketing and Impact.* Ann Arbor: Health Administration Press. 1985.

American Hospital Association. *Hospital Statistics*, 1980 Edition. Data from the AHA Annual Survey. Chicago: AHA. 1980.

Fleming, Gretchen V. and Ronald Andersen. *The Municipal Health Services Program: Can Access Be Improved While Controlling Costs?* Chicago: Pluribus Press, Inc. 1986.

Louis Harris and Associates. *Health Care for the Poor in Arizona.* New York: Louis Harris and Associates. 1983.

U.S. Department of Commerce, Bureau of Health Professions, National Technical Information Service. *Area Resource Files.* Springfield, VA: Office of Data Analysis and Management, Bureau of Health Professions. 1984.

Appendix B
Standard Errors of Estimates

CHRISTOPHER S. LYTTLE

THE SAMPLES for the five surveys analyzed here each represent one of a great number of potential samples that might have been drawn using the same universes, sample sizes, and designs. Each of these samples would have been somewhat different from all other potential samples, and so would have yielded slightly different estimates. Sampling error is the variance of a particular sample estimate from the mean of all possible sample estimates. The standard error of a survey estimate is a measure of the variation among the possible sample estimates, and is, therefore, an indicator of how precisely an estimate approximates the mean of potential samples.

One of the important uses of standard errors is the calculation of confidence intervals around a sample estimate. This is a measure of the probability that the mean of all possible sample estimates would fall within an interval. It is, for example, approximately 68 percent certain that the mean of all possible estimates would fall in the interval between one standard error above and one standard error below the obtained sample estimate. Similarly, the 90 percent confidence interval is between 1.6 standard errors below and 1.6 standard errors above the sample estimate; and plus or minus two standard errors yields a 95 percent confidence interval.

The error of a sample estimate may be decomposed into bias and variable error; and variable error may in turn be divided into sampling and nonsampling error. Andersen, et al. (1979) note that standard errors represent the sampling and part of the nonsampling components of total survey error. Bias results from a number of different sources, and so is controlled with different methods (stringent frame definitions, procedural controls, and appropriate nonsampling and nonresponse weights). These are assumed to be nonrandom errors, and are not corrected by the use of standard errors.

Discussions of standard errors for some studies may also be found elsewhere: for the 1982 National Access Survey, Appendix B in Aday, et al. (1984); for the Community Hospital Program (CHP) evaluation survey, Appendix B in Aday, et al. (1985); and for the Municipal Health Services Program (MHSP) evaluation survey, Appendix A in Fleming and Andersen (1986).

Calculation of Standard Errors

Traditionally, standard errors for large, complex surveys are computed by multiplying two components: a simple random sample standard error and a design factor. The design factors represent the deviation of the survey design from a completely random sampling process (Sudman, 1976). Typically, design factors are computed for a sample of estimates and generalized. Here they have been computed for a sample of estimates for the national, CHP and MHSP studies. Values for the Arizona and New York City surveys have been extrapolated from the other three surveys. Table B.1. shows these values grouped by variable type and sample subset. The variables used in the analysis that show high within family covariance include the following: family income, race, regular source of care, insurance, and residence. Examples of variables that show a low to medium within family covariance are age, sex, and hospitalizations.

Standard Errors of Percents

The standard error of a percent is calculated by multiplying the simple standard error of the percent by the design factor. The simple standard error of a percent is obtained by multiplying the percent and the quantity 100 minus the percent, divided by the unweighted number of cases, and taking the square root of the resultant estimate. For the convenience of the reader, Table B.2. contains a selected set of these values.

Example:

Table 5.1. shows that 52 percent of the cases in the national sample are female. The within-family covariance of sex is low, and this figure is for the whole sample (n = 6610) rather than one of the groups defined as above or below 150 percent of the poverty level. Therefore, the design factor selected from Table B.1. is 1.35. The simple random standard error from Table B.2. is 0.65 (at the intersection of 50 percent and a sample size of 6000). The standard error is the product of the design factor and the standard error (1.35 × 0.65 = 0.8775).

Standard Errors of Differences

The standard error of a difference between two estimates (σ_{A-B}) is dependent on the standard errors of the estimates (σ_A and σ_B), and the correlation between the components (ρ). It may be computed using the formula:

$$\sigma_{A-B} = (\sigma_A^2 + \sigma_B^2 - 2\rho\sigma_A\sigma_B)^{1/2}$$

If A or B is a subclass of the other then ρ is one. Otherwise using ρ equal to zero will yield an estimate that is only slightly high.

Example:

We have already seen that 52 percent of the cases for the national sample are female, with a standard error of 0.8775. In the Arizona sample 58 percent of the cases are female. The Arizona standard error is computed in the same fashion as for the national estimate: the product of the low within-family covariance design factor (1.15) and the simple random probability standard error for an estimate of about 60 percent and a sample size of about 3500 (0.83), or 0.9545. Since the Arizona sample is not a subset of the national sample, the standard error of the 6 percent difference between the national and Arizona samples is:

$$\sigma_{A-B} = (0.8775^2 + 0.9545^2)^{1/2} = 1.2966.$$

The 95 percent confidence interval is between 6 – (1.3 × 2) = 3.4 and 6 + (1.3 × 2) = 8.6. We may, therefore, say with 95 percent confidence that the proportion of women below poverty level in

Arizona is between 3.4 and 8.6 percent higher than in the country as a whole.

Standard Errors of Means

The sampling distribution of a mean, and therefore the standard error of a mean, reflects not only the number of cases in the sample, but also the shape of the variable's distribution. Tables B.3. and B.4. give standard errors for the means presented in Chapters 6 and 7. In calculating values for these tables, we adopted the rather conservative approach of using the weighted sums of squares and the unweighted number of cases, and then multiplying the simple standard error by the design factor. The formula is:

$$\text{Standard Error} = \text{Design Factor} \times (\Sigma_i W_i (X_i - \bar{X}_w)^2 / (N-1)N)^{1/2},$$

where W_i is the case weight, $\bar{X}_w$ is the weighted mean value of the variable, X_i is the case value on the variable, and N is the unweighted number of cases.

Standard Errors of Ratios

The standard error of a ratio ($\sigma_{A/B}$) is a functiaon of the components of the ratio (A and B), the standard errors of the components (σ_A and σ_B), and the correlation between the components (ρ). It may be computed with the formula:

$$\sigma_{A/B} = (A/B) \times ((\sigma_A/A)^2 + (\sigma_B/B)^2 - 2\rho\sigma_A\sigma_B/AB).^{1/2}$$

Table B.5. shows standard errors computed for ratios presented in Chapter 7. For these calculations the correlation between A and B was estimated to be .55 for emergency room and outpatient department to total ambulatory use, .96 for hospital use to total use, and .31 for the use to disability ratio.

Table B.1. Design Factors.

<u>1982 National Access Survey</u>:

    High within family covariance:

Less than 1.5 poverty	2.44
1.5 poverty or above	1.28
Other groups	1.69

    Low or medium within family covariance:

Less than 1.5 poverty	1.70
1.5 poverty or above	1.15
Other groups	1.35

<u>Arizona Low Income</u>:

High within family covariance:	1.28
Low or medium within family covariance:	1.15

<u>Community Hospital Program (CHP)</u>:

    Area Sample:

High within family covariance:	1.39
Medium within family covariance:	1.27
Low within family covariance:	1.05

List Sample:	1.00

<u>Municipal Health Services Program (MHSP)</u>:

High within family covariance:	1.94
Low or medium within family covariance:	1.50

<u>New York City</u>:

    High within family covariance:

Less than 1.5 poverty	2.44
1.5 poverty or above	1.28
Other groups	1.69

    Low or medium within family covariance:

Less than 1.5 poverty	1.70
1.5 poverty or above	1.15
Other groups	1.35

Table B.2. Simple Random Standard Errors of a Percent.*

PERCENT

SAMPLE SIZE	5 / 95	10 / 90	15 / 85	20 / 80	25 / 75	30 / 70	35 / 65	40 / 60	45 / 55	50 / 50
25	4.36	6.00	7.14	8.00	8.66	9.17	9.54	9.80	9.95	10.00
50	3.08	4.24	5.05	5.66	6.12	6.48	6.75	6.93	7.04	7.07
75	2.52	3.46	4.12	4.62	5.00	5.29	5.51	5.66	5.74	5.77
100	2.18	3.00	3.57	4.00	4.33	4.58	4.77	4.90	4.97	5.00
150	1.78	2.45	2.92	3.27	3.54	3.74	3.89	4.00	4.06	4.08
200	1.54	2.12	2.52	2.83	3.06	3.24	3.37	3.46	3.52	3.54
250	1.38	1.90	2.26	2.53	2.74	2.90	3.02	3.10	3.15	3.16
300	1.26	1.73	2.06	2.31	2.50	2.65	2.75	2.83	2.87	2.89
350	1.16	1.60	1.91	2.14	2.31	2.45	2.55	2.62	2.66	2.67
400	1.09	1.50	1.79	2.00	2.17	2.29	2.38	2.45	2.49	2.50
450	1.03	1.41	1.68	1.89	2.04	2.16	2.25	2.31	2.35	2.36
500	.97	1.34	1.60	1.79	1.94	2.05	2.13	2.19	2.22	2.24
600	.89	1.22	1.46	1.63	1.77	1.87	1.95	2.00	2.03	2.04
700	.82	1.13	1.35	1.51	1.64	1.73	1.80	1.85	1.88	1.89
800	.77	1.06	1.26	1.41	1.53	1.62	1.69	1.73	1.76	1.77
900	.73	1.00	1.19	1.33	1.44	1.53	1.59	1.63	1.66	1.67
1000	.69	.95	1.13	1.26	1.37	1.45	1.51	1.55	1.57	1.58
1500	.56	.77	.92	1.03	1.12	1.18	1.23	1.26	1.28	1.29
2000	.49	.67	.80	.89	.97	1.02	1.07	1.10	1.11	1.12
2500	.44	.60	.71	.80	.87	.92	.95	.98	.99	1.00
3000	.40	.55	.65	.73	.79	.84	.87	.89	.91	.91
3500	.37	.51	.60	.68	.73	.77	.81	.83	.84	.85
4000	.34	.47	.56	.63	.68	.72	.75	.77	.79	.79
4500	.32	.45	.53	.60	.65	.68	.71	.73	.74	.75
5000	.31	.42	.50	.57	.61	.65	.67	.69	.70	.71
6000	.28	.39	.46	.52	.56	.59	.62	.63	.64	.65
7000	.26	.36	.43	.48	.52	.55	.57	.59	.59	.60
8000	.24	.34	.40	.45	.48	.51	.53	.55	.56	.56
9000	.23	.32	.38	.42	.46	.48	.50	.52	.52	.53
10000	.22	.30	.36	.40	.43	.46	.48	.49	.50	.50
11000	.21	.29	.34	.38	.41	.44	.45	.47	.47	.48
12000	.20	.27	.33	.37	.40	.42	.44	.45	.45	.46
13000	.19	.26	.31	.35	.38	.40	.42	.43	.44	.44

* $(P (100 - P) / N)^{1/2}$

Table B.3. Standard Error of Means, Chapter 6.

INSURANCE COVERAGE

DATA SETS	Whole Data Set	Public Only	Private Only	Public and Private	None
			Design Factors		
1982 National	1.35	1.69	1.69	1.69	1.69
Arizona Low Income	1.15	1.28	1.28	1.28	1.28
CHP	1.05	1.39	1.39	1.39	1.39
MHSP	1.50	1.94	1.94	1.94	1.94
New York City	1.35	1.69	1.69	1.69	1.69
			Standard Errors		
Non-hospital Disability Days					
1982 National	3.06	12.93	3.56	15.70	6.56
Arizona Low Income	2.82	6.86	4.72	10.51	4.70
CHP	7.67	40.37	9.46	59.27	25.72
MHSP	8.15	29.42	10.36	57.16	18.84
New York City	1.89	6.36	2.69	8.87	4.41
Number of Symptoms					
CHP	0.31	1.27	0.44	1.93	1.42
MHSP	0.25	0.87	0.38	1.27	0.65
Mean Severity of Symptoms					
CHP	0.19	0.78	0.26	1.23	0.83
MHSP	0.15	0.54	0.23	0.81	0.39

Table B.3. Standard Error of Means, Chapter 6 (continued).

REGULAR SOURCE OF CARE

DATA SETS	Private Office/ Clinic	Hospital OPD	Hospital ER	Other	No Regular Source
			Design Factors		
1982 National	1.69	1.69	1.69	1.69	1.69
Arizona Low Income	1.28	1.28	1.28	1.28	1.28
CHP	1.39	1.39	1.39	1.39	1.39
MHSP	1.94	1.94	1.94	1.94	1.94
New York City	1.69	1.69	1.69	1.69	1.69
			Standard Errors		
Non-hospital Disability Days					
1982 National	4.52	18.27	38.73	11.64	7.44
Arizona Low Income	5.17	6.32	20.23	7.76	6.48
CHP	12.29	49.45	66.72	49.21	14.85
MHSP	16.60	35.16	32.96	18.01	19.09
New York City	3.24	7.27	10.60	6.62	4.15
Number of Symptoms					
CHP	0.48	1.93	2.25	2.15	0.98
MHSP	0.49	1.02	1.19	0.61	0.72
Mean Severity of Symptoms					
CHP	0.29	1.18	1.33	1.37	0.58
MHSP	0.30	0.63	0.70	0.37	0.42

Table B.4. Standard Error of Means, Chapter 7 - 1982 National Survey

ANALYTIC GROUPS	Design Factors	Waiting Time	Physician Visits	Hospital Days
Whole data set	1.35	2.93	.54	2.25
Insurance Coverage				
Public Only	1.69	8.93	2.03	3.07
Private Only	1.69	5.16	.86	4.52
Public and Private	1.69	7.26	1.73	5.48
No Insurance	1.69	8.76	1.45	9.11
Regular Source				
Private Office/Clinic	1.69	3.42	.83	2.87
Hospital OPD	1.69	25.15	2.65	8.47
Hospital ER	1.69	37.86	2.71	51.22
Other Source	1.69	12.36	1.74	13.52
No Regular Source	1.69	12.08	1.27	6.94
Race				
White	1.69	2.84	.56	2.46
Black	1.69	13.01	1.71	8.62
Hispanic	1.69	15.26	1.95	3.15
Poverty Level				
Less Than Poverty	1.70	5.20	1.14	3.03
1.0-1.5 Poverty	1.70	3.03	.69	1.74
Greater Than 1.5	1.15	5.30	.86	6.09

Table B.5. Standard Error of Ratios, Chapter 7 - 1982 National Survey.

ANALYTIC GROUPS	Design Factors	Inpatient All Visits	Disability MD Visits	ER & OPD MD Visits
Whole Data Set	1.35	.31	.60	.03
Insurance Coverage				
Public Only	1.69	.28	1.65	.07
Private Only	1.69	.71	.76	.05
Public and Private	1.69	.32	2.52	.07
No Insurance	1.69	2.89	1.48	.11
Regular Source				
Private Office/Clinic	1.69	.43	.88	.04
Hospital OPD	1.69	.90	2.76	.19
Hospital ER	1.69	.65	8.58	.28
Other Source	1.69	1.61	2.04	.07
No Regular Source	1.69	3.59	2.50	.18
Race				
White	1.69	.42	.87	.04
Black	1.69	1.16	2.49	.14
Hispanic	1.69	1.41	1.78	.09
Poverty Level				
Less Than Poverty	1.70	.41	1.14	.07
1.0-1.5 Poverty	1.70	.12	.58	.03
Greater Than 1.5	1.15	.73	1.07	.05

References

Aday, Lu Ann, et al. *Access to Medical Care in the U.S.: Who Has it, Who Doesn't.* Chicago: Pluribus Press, Inc. 1984.

Aday, Lu Ann, et al. *Hospital-Physician Sponsored Primary Care: Marketing and Impact.* Ann Arbor: Health Administration Press. 1985.

Andersen, Ronald M., et al. *Total Survey Error.* San Francisco, CA: Jossey-Bass. 1979.

Fleming, Gretchen V. and Ronald Andersen. *The Municipal Health Services Program: Can Access Be Improved While Controlling Costs?* Chicago: Pluribus Press, Inc. 1986.

Sudman, Seymour *Applied Sampling.* New York: Academic Press, Inc. 1976.

References

Aday, Lu Ann and Ronald Andersen. "A Framework for the Study of Access to Medical Care." *Health Services Research* 9 (Fall 1974): 208–220.

Aday, Lu Ann and Ronald Andersen. *Development of Indices of Access to Medical Care*. Ann Arbor: Health Administration Press. 1975.

Aday, Lu Ann and Ronald Andersen. "Equity of Access to Medical Care: A Conceptual and Empirical Overview." *Medical Care* 19 (December 1981 Supplement): 4–27.

Aday, Lu Ann, et al. *Health Care in the U.S.: Equitable for Whom?* Beverly Hills: Sage Publications. 1980.

Aday, Lu Ann, et al. *Access to Medical Care in the U.S.: Who Has it, Who Doesn't*. Chicago: Pluribus Press, Inc. 1984.

Aday, Lu Ann, et al. *Hospital-Physician Sponsored Primary Care: Marketing and Impact*. Ann Arbor: Health Administration Press. 1985.

Altman, Drew. "Health Care for the Poor." *Annals of the American Academy of Political and Social Sciences* 468 (July 1983): 103–121.

American Medical Association. *Physician Characteristics and Distribution in the U.S.* Chicago: AMA. 1985.

American Public Health Association. "The 1986 President's Budget." *The Nation's Health* (March 1985): 6–13.

Andersen, Ronald. *A Behavioral Model of Families' Use of Health Services*. Research Series No. 25. Chicago: Center for Health Administration Studies, The University of Chicago. 1968.

Andersen, Ronald, et al. *Equity in Health Services: Empirical Analyses in Social Policy.* Cambridge, MA: Ballinger. 1975.

Andersen, Ronald, et al. *Two Decades of Health Services: Social Survey Trends in Use and Expenditure.* Cambridge, MA: Ballinger. 1976.

Andersen, Ronald and Lu Ann Aday. "Access to Medical Care in the U.S.: Realized and Potential." *Medical Care* 16 (July 1978): 533–546.

Andersen, Ronald, et al. *Total Survey Error.* San Francisco, CA: Jossey-Bass. 1979.

Anderson, Odin W. "Health Services in the United States: A Growth Enterprise for a Hundred Years." In T. J. Litman and L. S. Robins (eds.), *Health Politics and Policy.* New York: John Wiley and Sons (1984): 67–79.

Anderson, Odin W. *Health Services in the United States: A Growth Enterprise Since 1875.* Ann Arbor: Health Administration Press. 1985.

Anderson, Odin W. and Norman Gevitz. "The General Hospital: A Social and Historical Perspective." In D. Mechanic (ed.), *Handbook of Health, Health Care, and the Health Professions.* New York: The Free Press (1983): 305–317.

Berki, Sylvester E. and Marie L. Ashcraft. "On the Analysis of Ambulatory Utilization: An Investigation of the Roles of Need, Access and Price as Predictors of Illness and Preventive Visits." *Medical Care* 17 (December, 1979): 1163–1181.

Berki, Sylvester E., et al. "Health Insurance Coverage of the Unemployed." *Medical Care* 23 (July 1985): 847–854.

Bryant, John H., et al. *Community Hospitals and Primary Care.* Cambridge, MA: Ballinger. 1976.

Cafferata, Gail Lee. "Knowledge of Their Health Insurance Coverage by the Elderly." *Medical Care* 22 (September 1984): 835–847.

Cafferata, Gail Lee. "Private Health Insurance of the Medicare Population and the Baucus Legislation." *Medical Care* 23 (September 1985): 1086–1096.

Cleary, Paul D. and Alan M. Jette. "The Validity of Self-Reported Physician Utilization Measures." *Medical Care* 22 (September 1984): 796–803.

Committee on the Costs of Medical Care. *Medical Care for the American People: The Final Report on the Committee on the Costs of Medical Care.* Chicago: University of Chicago Press. 1932.

Congressional Budget Office. *Changing the Structure of Medicare Benefits: Issues and Options.* Washington, D.C.: Congressional Budget Office. 1983.

Congressional Quarterly. (14 December 1985): 2609–2611.

Council on Research and Development, American Hospital Association. "Health Care for the Indigent: Research Agenda for the Future." *Health Services Research* 21 (August 1986): 395–401.

Crandall, Lee A. and R. Paul Duncan. "Attitudinal and Situational Factors in the Use of Physician Services by Low-Income Persons." *Journal of Health and Social Behavior* 22 (March 1981): 64–77.

Davidson, Stephen M. "Understanding the Growth of Emergency Department Utilization." *Medical Care* 16 (February 1978): 122–132.

Davis, Karen and Diane Rowland. "Uninsured and Underserved: Inequities in Health Care in the United States." *Milbank Memorial Fund Quarterly* 61 (Spring 1983): 149–176.

Dolenc, Danielle and Charles J. Dougherty. "DRGs: the Counterrevolution in Financing Health Care." *Hastings Center Report* 15 (June 1985): 19–29.

Duan, Naihua, et al. "A Comparison of Alternative Models for the Demand for Medical Care." *Journal of Business and Economic Statistics* 1 (1983): 115–126.

Enthoven, Alain C. "The Rand Experiment and Economical Health Care." *New England Journal of Medicine* 310 (7 June 1984): 1528–1530.

Falk, Isidore Sydney, et al. *The Costs of Medical Care: A Summary of Investigations on the Economic Aspects of the Prevention and Care of Illness.* Chicago: University of Chicago Press. 1933.

Feder, Judith, et al. "Falling Through the Cracks: Poverty, Insurance Coverage, and Hospital Care for the Poor, 1980 and 1982." *Milbank Memorial Fund Quarterly/Health and Society* 62 (Fall 1984): 544–566.

Fleming, Gretchen V. and Ronald Andersen. *The Municipal Health Services Program: Can Access Be Improved While Controlling Costs?* Chicago: Pluribus Press, Inc. 1986.

Flinn Foundation. *Health Care for Arizona's Poor, 1982–84.* Phoenix: Flinn Foundation. 1985.

Freeman, Howard E. and Bradford Kirkman-Liff. "Health Care Under AHCCCS: An Examination of Arizona's Alternative to Medicaid." *Health Services Research* 30 (August 1985): 245–266.

Freeman, Howard E. and Hye Kyung Lee. "New Yorkers' Perceptions of their Health Care." Unpublished manuscript. Los Angeles: Department of Sociology, UCLA. 1984.

Gabel, Jon R. and Thomas H. Rice. "Reducing Public Expenditures for Physicians: The Price of Paying Less." *Journal of Health Politics, Policy and Law* 9 (Winter 1985): 595–609.

Goldberg, Harold I. and Allen J. Dietrich. "The Continuity of Care Provided to Primary Care Patients. A Comparison of Family Physicians, General Internists and Medical Subspecialists." *Medical Care* 23 (January 1985): 63–73.

Goldsmith, Jeff Charles. *Can Hospitals Survive? The New Competitive Market.* Homewood, IL: Dow Jones-Irwin. 1981.

Goldsmith, Seth B. *Ambulatory Care.* Germantown, MD: Aspen Systems Corporation. 1977.

Gortmaker, Steven L. "Medicaid and the Health Care of Children in Poverty and

Near Poverty. Some Successes and Failures." *Medical Care* 19 (June 1981): 567–582.

Graduate Medical Education Advisory Committee (GMENAC) *Summary Report, Volume I.* DHHS Publication No. (HRA) 81–651. Washington, DC: Public Health Service. 1981.

Hartwell, R. M. "The Economic History of Medical Care." In M. Perlman (ed.), *Economics of Health and Medical Care.* New York: Cromwell, Collier, and Macmillan (1975): 3–38.

Health Care Financing Administration. Unpublished data. Office of Statistical Information Services, Building 1A-15, 6325 Security Blvd., Baltimore, MD 21207. 1986.

Health Care Financing Administration. Unpublished data. Office of the Actuary, Building 1A-15, 6325 Security Blvd., Baltimore, MD 21207. 1987.

Health Care Financial Management. 40 (February 1986): 5–7.

Health Care Financing Review. 6 (Spring 1985): Table 8.

Hershey, John C., et al. "Making Sense Out of Utilization Data." *Medical Care* 13 (October 1975): 838–54.

Iglehart, John K. "Medical Care of the Poor—A Growing Problem." *New England Journal of Medicine* 313 (4 July 1985): 59–63.

Iglehart, John K. "Health Policy Report: Federal Support of Health Manpower Education." *New England Journal of Medicine* 312 (23 May 1986): 1400–1404.

Jacobs, Arthur R. and Christine L. Thurber. "Emergency Care Crisis Avoided in a Rural Community." *Health Services Reports* 87 (December 1972): 977–982.

Kasper, Judith A. and Gerald Barrish. "Usual Sources of Medical Care and Their Characteristics." *National Medical Care Expenditures Study.* Data Preview 12. Hyattsville, MD: National Center for Health Services Research. 1982.

Keith, Stephen N., et al. "Effects of Affirmative Action in Medical Schools: A Study of the Class of 1975." *New England Journal of Medicine* 313 (12 December 1985): 1519–1525.

Kohn, Robert and Kerr L. White. *Health Care—An International Study: Report of the World Health Organization/International Collaborative Study of Medical Care Utilization.* London: Oxford University Press. 1976.

Kirkman-Liff, Bradford L. "Profile of the Chronically Ill Indigent Population in Arizona Prior to AHCCCS." HS 83/84:1. Tempe: Center for Health Services Administration, Arizona State University. 1984a.

Kirkman-Liff, Bradford L. "A Comparison of Access and Satisfaction With Health Care Between Arizona Indigents and Total United States Population." HS 83/84:2. Tempe: Center for Health Services Administration, Arizona State University. 1984b.

Kirkman-Liff, Bradford L., et al. *Analysis of Indigent Health Care Data for*

Maricopa County, Arizona. Final Report to the Flinn Foundation. Tempe: Center for Health Services Administration, Arizona State University. 1982.

Kosecoff, Jacqueline, et al. "General Medical Care and the Education of Internists in University Hospitals." *Annals of Internal Medicine* 102 (February 1985): 250–257.

Kuder, John M. and Gary S. Levitz. "Visits to the Physician: An Evaluation of the Usual-Source Effect." *Health Services Research* 20 (December 1985): 579–596.

Leiderman, Deborah and Jean-Anne Grisso. "The Gomer Phenomenon." *Journal of Health and Social Behavior* 26 (September 1985): 222–232.

Lerner, Monroe, et al. "The Decline in the Blue Cross Plan Admission Rate: Four Explanations." *Inquiry* 20 (Summer 1983): 103–113.

Lewis, Charles E., et al. *A Right to Health: The Problem of Access to Primary Medical Care.* New York: John Wiley and Sons, Inc. 1976.

Linn, Lawrence S., et al. "Physician and Patient Satisfaction as Factors Related to the Organization of Internal Medicine Group Practices." *Medical Care* 23 (October 1985): 1171–1178.

Lohr, Kathleen N. and M. Susan Marquis. *Medicare and Medicaid: Past, Present and Future.* Rand Report #N-2088-HHS/RC. Santa Monica, CA: Rand. 1984.

Louis Harris and Associates. *Access to Health Care Services in the United States: 1982.* New York: Louis Harris and Associates. 1982a.

Louis Harris and Associates. *Health Care in New York City.* New York: Louis Harris and Associates. 1982b.

Louis Harris and Associates. *Health Care for the Poor in Arizona.* New York: Louis Harris and Associates. 1983.

Luft, Harold S. *Health Maintenance Organizations: Dimensions of Performance.* New York: John Wiley & Sons, Inc. 1981.

Mahoney, Margaret E. "What New Yorkers Say About Their Health Care." *President's Essay: 1982 Annual Report of The Commonwealth Fund.* New York: Commonwealth Fund. 1982.

Marcus, Alfred C. and Jeffrey P. Stone. "Mode of Payment and Identification with a Regular Doctor. A Prospective Look at Reported Use of Services." *Medical Care* 22 (July 1984): 647–660.

Mechanic, David. "Correlates of Physician Utilization: Why Do Major Multivariate Studies of Physician Utilization Find Trivial Psychosocial and Organizational Effects?" *Journal of Health and Social Behavior* 20 (December 1979): 387–396.

Miller, Don M. "Reducing Transformation Bias in Curve Fitting." *The American Statistician* 38 (May 1984): 124–126.

Mitchell, Janet B. and Rachel Shurman. "Access to Private Obstetrics/

Gynecology Services Under Medicaid." *Medical Care* 22 (November 1984): 1026–37.

Morone, James A. and Andrew B. Dunham. "The Waning of Professional Dominance: DRGs and the Hospitals." *Health Affairs* 3 (Spring 1984): 73–87.

Mulstein, Suzanne. "The Uninsured and the Financing of Uncompensated Care: Scope, Costs and Policy Options." *Inquiry* 21 (Fall 1984): 214–229.

Mundinger, Mary O'Neil. "Health Service Funding Cuts and the Declining Health of the Poor." *New England Journal of Medicine* 313 (4 July 1985): 44–46.

National Center for Health Statistics. *Health, United States, 1984.* DHHS Publication No. (PHS) 84-1232. Washington, DC: U.S. Government Printing Office, 1984.

National Center for Health Statistics. *Health, United States, 1985.* DHHS Publication No. (PHS) 85-1232. Washington, DC: U.S. Government Printing Office. 1985.

Newcomer, Robert, et al. "Medicare Prospective Payment: Anticipated Effect on Hospitals, Other Community Agencies, and Families." *Journal of Health Politics, Policy and Law* 10 (Summer 1985): 275–282.

Newhouse, Joseph P., et al. "Some Interim Results From a Controlled Trial of Cost Sharing in Health Insurance." *New England Journal of Medicine* 305 (17 December 1981): 1501–7.

Okada, Louise M. and Thomas T. H. Wan. "Medicaid, Medicare, and Private Insurance Coverage in Five Urban Areas." *Inquiry* 15 (December 1978): 336–344.

President's Commission for the Study of Ethical Problems in Medicine and Biomedical and Behavioral Research. *Securing Access to Health Care: The Ethical Implications of Differences in the Availability of Health Services. Volume I: Report.* Washington, D.C.: U.S. Government Printing Office. 1983.

Rosenberg, Charles E. "From Almshouse to Hospital: The Shaping of Philadelphia General Hospital." *Milbank Memorial Fund Quarterly* 60 (Winter 1982): 108–54.

Roth, Julius A. "Utilization of the Hospital Emergency Department." *Journal of Health and Social Behavior* 12 (December 1971): 312–320.

Schiff, Robert L., et al. "Transfers to a Public Hospital: A Prospective Study of 467 Patients." *New England Journal of Medicine* 314 (27 February 1986): 552–557.

Schneider, Karen C. and Henry G. Dove. "High Users of VA Emergency Room Facilities: Are Outpatients Abusing the System or Is the System Abusing Them?" *Inquiry* 20 (Spring 1983): 57–64.

Sharp, Kenneth, et al. "Symptoms, Beliefs, and the Use of Physician Services Among the Disadvantaged." *Journal of Health and Social Behavior* 24 (September 1983): 255–263.

Shea, Steven and Mindy Thompson Fullilove. "Entry of Black and Other Minority Students into U.S. Medical Schools: Historical Perspectives and Recent Trends." *New England Journal of Medicine* 313 (10 October 1985): 933–940.

Shortell, Stephen M., et al. *Hospital Physician Joint Ventures: Results and Lessons from a National Demonstration.* Ann Arbor, MI: Health Administration Press. 1984.

Sloan, Frank A., et al. (ed.). *Uncompensated Hospital Care: Rights and Responsibilities.* Baltimore: Johns Hopkins Press. 1986.

Spiegel, Allen D. and Florence Kavaler. "The Debate Over Diagnosis Related Groups." *Journal of Community Health* 10 (Summer 1985): 81–92.

Starr, Paul. *The Social Transformation of American Medicine: The Rise of a Sovereign Profession and the Making of a Vast Industry.* New York: Basic Books Incorporated. 1982.

Stratmann, William D. and Ralph Ullman. "A Study of Consumer Attitudes about Health Care: The Role of the Emergency Room." *Medical Care* 13 (December 1975): 1033–1043.

Straus, John H., et al. "Referrals from an Emergency Room to Primary Care Practices at an Urban Hospital." *American Journal of Public Health* 73 (January 1983): 57–61.

Stuart, Bruce et al. "Medicaid Reform: Programming Solutions to the Equity Problem." *Journal of Health Politics, Policy and Law* 10 (Spring 1985): 93–118.

Thompson, Frank J. *Health Policy and the Bureaucracy: Politics and Implementation.* Cambridge, MA: The MIT Press. 1981.

Ullman, Ralph, et al. "An Emergency Room's Patients: Their Characteristics and Utilization of Hospital Services." *Medical Care* 13 (December 1975): 1011–1020.

U.S. Department of Commerce, Bureau of the Census. *Statistical Abstract of the United States, 1985.* Washington, D.C.: U.S. Government Printing Office (1985): Table 157.

U.S. Department of Commerce, Bureau of the Census. Unpublished data. Population Division, Washington, D.C. 20233. 1986.

U.S. Department of Commerce, Bureau of Health Professions, National Technical Information Service. *Area Resource Files.* Springfield, VA: Office of Data Analysis and Management, Bureau of Health Professions. 1984.

U.S. Department of Health Education and Welfare. "History and Evolution of Medicaid." In A.D. Spiegel and S. Podair (eds.), *Medicaid: Lessons for National Health Insurance.* Rockville, MD: Aspen Systems Corporation. 1975.

Walden, Daniel C., et al. "Changes in Health Insurance Status: Full-Year and Part-Year Coverage." *National Center for Health Services Research.* Rockville, MD (1985): 3–15.

Wan, Thomas T. H. "Use of Health Services by the Elderly in Low-Income Communities." *Milbank Memorial Fund Quarterly/Health and Society* 60 (Winter 1982): 82–107.

Wan, Thomas T. H. and Lois C. Gray. "Differential Access to Preventive Services for Children in Low Income Urban Areas." *Journal of Health and Social Behavior* 19 (September 1978): 312–324.

White, H. A. and P. A. O'Connor. "Use of the Emergency Room in a Community Hospital." *Public Health Reports* 85 (February 1970): 163–168.

Wilensky, Gail R. and Louis F. Rossiter. "The Relative Importance of Physician-Induced Demand in the Demand for Medical Care." *Milbank Memorial Fund Quarterly/Health and Society* 61 (Winter 1983): 252–277.

Wilensky, Gail, et al. "Variations in Health Insurance Coverage: Benefits vs. Premiums." *Milbank Memorial Fund Quarterly/Health and Society* 62 (Winter 1984): 53–81.

Williams, Stephen J. "Ambulatory Health Care Services." In S.J. Williams and P.R. Torrens (eds.), *Introduction to Health Services (2nd. ed.).* New York: John Wiley & Sons (1984): 135–171.

Wolinsky, Fredric D. "Assessing the Effects of Predisposing, Enabling, and Illness-Morbidity Characteristics on Health Service Utilization." *Journal of Health and Social Behavior* 19 (December 1978): 384–396.

Yelin, Edward H., et al. "Is Health Care Use Equivalent Across Social Groups? A Diagnosis-Based Study." *American Journal of Public Health* 73 (May 1983): 563–71.

Index